BREAST CANCER SCREENING AND PREVENTION

CANCER ETIOLOGY, DIAGNOSIS AND TREATMENTS

Additional books in this series can be found on Nova's website under the Series tab.

Additional E-books in this series can be found on Nova's website under the E-books tab.

CANCER ETIOLOGY, DIAGNOSIS AND TREATMENTS

BREAST CANCER SCREENING AND PREVENTION

JONATHAN D. PEGG
EDITOR

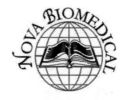

Nova Science Publishers, Inc.
New York

LIBRARY OF CONGRESS CATALOGING-IN-PUBLICATION DATA

Breast cancer screening and prevention / editor, Jonathan D. Pegg.
   p. ; cm.
Includes bibliographical references and index.
ISBN 978-1-61209-288-1 (softcover)
1. Breast--Cancer--Diagnosis. 2. Breast--Cancer--Prevention. I. Pegg, Jonathan D.
[DNLM: 1. Breast Neoplasms--diagnosis. 2. Breast Neoplasms--prevention & control. WP 870]
RC280.B8B6882 2011
616.99'449075--dc23
           2011022174

Published by Nova Science Publishers, Inc. † New York

CONTENTS

PREFACE

This book presents and discusses research in the study of breast cancer diagnosis and prevention. Topics discussed include strategies for the prevention of breast cancer; health benefits and breast cancer screenings; access to mammography facilities; the reduction in the risk of human breast cancer by selective cyclooxygenase-2 (COX-2) inhibitors and breast cancer perceptions and knowledge among women living in a rural community.

Chapter 1 - The epidemiology of breast cancer has focussed mainly on endogenous and exogenous endocrine risk factors for the disease. The picture emerging is that the greater the number of menstrual cycles to which the mammary epithelium is exposed, the higher the risk of breast cancer. Late menarche is protective as is early menopause and lactation. One paradox is the impact of age at first baby: this is protective up to age 30, but beyond that leads to an increased risk. Oophorectomy before the age of 35 leads to a two thirds reduction in risk of breast cancer but at the cost of severe menopausal symptoms and greater likelihood of osteoporosis. Another paradox is that ovarian ablation in BRCA1 carriers leads to a substantial lowering of risk of breast cancer, even though the phenotype of tumours in this group is usually ER/PR negative.

The major prevention studies have used selective estrogen receptor modulators (SERMS) with the aim of inhibiting estrogen uptake by breast epithelium and have shown a halving of risk and in the IBIS trial this effect was maintained during the 5 years after Tamoxifen had been stopped. In the MORE trial, Raloxifene reduced the incidence of breast cancer by 65% but as in IBIS and NSABP P1 trials the effect was restricted to ER+ve tumours: no reduction in ER-ve cancers was seen.

Life-style factors such as diet, obesity and exercise have a mild to moderate impact on risk but it is at present unlikely that these will have widespread application. Similarly, reduction of alcohol intake could lead to a modest reduction in the risk of breast cancer but possibly adversely affect cardiovascular diseases and would not be acceptable to the majority of the population. A long-term study of fenretinide in breast cancer patients has shown a 50% reduction in risk of second primaries in women aged ≤40 years.

As well as oophorectomy, bilateral prophylactic mastectomy has been found to reduce risk in a non-randomised trial for women with *BRCA1/2* mutations. In the future, selective ablation of mammary epithelium with conservation of stromal tissue may obviate the need for surgery. Trials are underway using aromatase inhibitors but these will only be applicable to postmenopausal women. Other potentially useful agents include new generation SERMs, demethylating agents, non-selective COX inhibitors, tyrosine kinase inhibitors and polyamine synthesis inhibitors. As our knowledge of non-endocrine risk factors increases so new interventions will emerge to reduce the incidence of both ER+ve and ER-ve breast cancer.

Chapter 2 - This research analyzes the beliefs and attitudes towards breast cancer and mammography –using the sociocognitive postulated by the health beliefs models- associated with different stages of mammography adoption. A cross-sectional design was used. The sample was consisting of Spanish women (N= 151), aged 47-70 years. They were evaluated by the same questionnaire, which measured two types of variables: (i) Socio-cognitive: perceived severity of breast cancer, perceived susceptibility to breast cancer, general health motivation, benefits and barriers perceived to mammography, social pressure, perceived control on this preventive behaviour and the degree of information about breast cancer screening; and (ii) Stage of mammography adoption: Precontemplation, Contemplation, Action, Action-Maintenance and Relapse. All the cognitive variables, except the perceived susceptibility to breast cancer, have significant differences depending on the stage of mammography adoption. According to the stages of adoption, the women differ as for their beliefs towards mammography screening and breast cancer, differ also in the control and social pressure that they perceive to undergo mammograms, and in the degree of information that they have about breast cancer screening mammography. The results of this research may inform interventions to increase mammography use.

Chapter 3 – The authors performed this study to assess women's perceptions, knowledge and behavioral practices for breast cancer prevention in a rural setting. A 61-item questionnaire was developed based on Health

Belief Model constructs and completed by 185 women age 35 and older. Results showed significant differences in several areas including perceived susceptibility and severity. Overall knowledge was poor. In logistic regression perceived barriers and yearly clinical breast examination appeared to be significant predictors for regular screening behavior (OR=0.02, CI=0.03-0.09 and OR=0.23, CI=0.05-0.99, respectively). Behavioral interventions targeting barriers for rural women need to be designed to include consideration of specific barriers and clear information on the need for regular screening.

Chapter 4 - *Objectives:* The objective of the study was to examine the association between access to mammography facilities and utilization of screening mammography in an urban population.

Methods: Data on female breast cancer cases were obtained from an extensive mammography surveillance project. Distance to mammography facilities was measured by using GIS, which was followed by measuring geographical access to mammography facilities using Floating Catchment Area (FCA) Method (considering all available facilities within an arbitrary radius from the woman's residence by using Arc GIS 9.0 software).

Results: Of 2,024 women, 91.4% were Caucasian; age ranged from 25 to 98 years; most (95%) were non-Hispanic in origin. Logistic regression found age, family history, hormone replacement therapy, physician recommendation, and breast cancer stage at diagnosis to be significant predictors of having had a previous mammogram. Women having higher access to mammography facilities were less likely to have had a previous mammogram compared to women who had low access, considering all the facilities within 10 miles (OR=0.41, CI=0.22-0.76), 30 miles (OR=0.52, CI=0.29-0.91) and 40 miles (OR=0.51, CI=0.28-0.92) radiuses. *Conclusions:* Physical distance to mammography facilities does not necessarily predict utilization of mammogram and greater access does not assure greater utilizations, due to constraints imposed by socio economic and cultural barriers. Future studies should focus on measuring access to mammography facilities capturing a broader dimension of access considering qualitative aspect of facilities, as well as other travel impedances.

Chapter 5 - This study examined the association between access to mammography facilities and breast cancer stage at diagnosis in an urban population. Data on female breast cancer cases were obtained from an extensive mammography surveillance project. The Floating Catchment Area Method, considering all available facilities within an arbitrary radius from woman's residence, was used to assess access to mammography facilities. Results showed that odds of breast cancer being diagnosed at an advanced stage were higher for women who had greater access compared to women who had lower access to mammogram facilities. Greater access did not assure breast cancer to be diagnosed at less advanced stage due to constraints imposed by socio economic and cultural barriers. Future studies should measure access to mammography facilities capturing a broader dimension of access.

Chapter 6 - Epidemiologic and laboratory investigations suggest that nonsteroidal anti-inflammatory drugs (NSAIDs) have chemopreventive effects against breast cancer due to their activity against cyclooxygenase-2 (COX-2), the rate-limiting enzyme of the prostaglandin cascade.

The authors conducted a case control study of breast cancer designed to compare effects of selective and non-selective COX-2 inhibitors. A total of 611 incident breast cancer patients were ascertained from the James Cancer Hospital, Columbus, Ohio, during 2003-2004 and compared with 615 cancer free controls frequency-matched to the cases on age, race, and county of residence. Data on the past and current use of prescription and over the counter medications and breast cancer risk factors were ascertained using a standardized risk factor questionnaire. Effects of COX-2 inhibiting agents were quantified by calculating odds ratios (OR) and 95% confidence intervals.

Results showed significant risk reductions for selective COX-2 inhibitors as a group (OR=0.15, 95% CI=0.08-0.28), regular aspirin (OR=0.46, 95% CI = 0.32-0.65), and ibuprofen or naproxen (0.36, 95% CI= 0.21-0.60). Intake of COX-2 inhibitors produced significant risk reductions for premenopausal women (OR=0.05), postmenopausal women (OR=0.26), women with a positive family history (OR=0.19), women with a negative family history (OR=0.14), women with estrogen receptor positive tumors (OR=0.24), women with estrogen receptor negative tumors (OR=0.05), women with HER-2/neu positive tumors (OR=0.26), and women with HER-2/neu negative tumors (OR=0.17). Acetaminophen, a compound with negligible COX-2 activity produced no significant change in the risk of breast cancer.

Selective COX-2 inhibitors (celecoxib and rofecoxib) were only recently approved for use in 1999, and rofecoxib (Vioxx) was withdrawn from the marketplace in 2004. Nevertheless, even in the short window of exposure to these compounds, the selective COX-2 inhibitors produced a significant (85%) reduction in the risk of breast cancer, underscoring their strong potential for breast cancer chemoprevention.

In: Breast Cancer Screening and Prevention   ISBN 978-1-61209-288-1
Editor: Jonathan D. Pegg   © 2011 Nova Science Publishers, Inc.

Chapter 1

STRATEGIES FOR PREVENTION
OF BREAST CANCER

*Ruchi Tandon and Ian S Fentiman**
Hedley Atkins Breast Unit, Guy's Hospital, London SE1 9RT

ABSTRACT

The epidemiology of breast cancer has focussed mainly on endogenous and exogenous endocrine risk factors for the disease. The picture emerging is that the greater the number of menstrual cycles to which the mammary epithelium is exposed, the higher the risk of breast cancer. Late menarche is protective as is early menopause and lactation. One paradox is the impact of age at first baby: this is protective up to age 30, but beyond that leads to an increased risk. Oophorectomy before the age of 35 leads to a two thirds reduction in risk of breast cancer but at the cost of severe menopausal symptoms and greater likelihood of osteoporosis. Another paradox is that ovarian ablation in BRCA1 carriers leads to a substantial lowering of risk of breast cancer, even though the phenotype of tumours in this group is usually ER/PR negative.

The major prevention studies have used selective estrogen receptor modulators (SERMS) with the aim of inhibiting estrogen uptake by breast epithelium and have shown a halving of risk and in the IBIS trial this

---

* Corresponding author: Ian.Fentiman@gstt.nhs. uk

effect was maintained during the 5 years after Tamoxifen had been stopped. In the MORE trial, Raloxifene reduced the incidence of breast cancer by 65% but as in IBIS and NSABP P1 trials the effect was restricted to ER+ve tumours: no reduction in ER-ve cancers was seen.

Life-style factors such as diet, obesity and exercise have a mild to moderate impact on risk but it is at present unlikely that these will have widespread application. Similarly, reduction of alcohol intake could lead to a modest reduction in the risk of breast cancer but possibly adversely affect cardiovascular diseases and would not be acceptable to the majority of the population. A long-term study of fenretinide in breast cancer patients has shown a 50% reduction in risk of second primaries in women aged ≤40 years.

As well as oophorectomy, bilateral prophylactic mastectomy has been found to reduce risk in a non-randomised trial for women with *BRCA1/2* mutations. In the future, selective ablation of mammary epithelium with conservation of stromal tissue may obviate the need for surgery. Trials are underway using aromatase inhibitors but these will only be applicable to postmenopausal women. Other potentially useful agents include new generation SERMs, demethylating agents, non-selective COX inhibitors, tyrosine kinase inhibitors and polyamine synthesis inhibitors. As our knowledge of non-endocrine risk factors increases so new interventions will emerge to reduce the incidence of both ER+ve and ER-ve breast cancer.

Keywords: breast cancer, prevention, tamoxifen, fenretinide, raloxifene, COX inhibitors

INTRODUCTION

Breast cancer is increasing in incidence such that it is now the most common cancer to affect women and is the second highest cause of their mortality (after lung cancer) [1]. It is estimated that a woman surviving to the age of 85 has a one in nine chance of developing breast cancer. The disease has identifiable risk factors so that some high-risk individuals can be identified and monitored in the hope of early detection. Risk factors include genetic mutations predisposing to inadequate DNA repair (BRCA1 and BRCA2) [2], age [3] and environmental influences that increase circulating levels of estrogen, early menarche, late menopause [4] late first childbirth [5], hormone replacement therapy [6, 7], and body mass index [8]. Other factors include, family history of breast cancer [9], abnormal breast biopsy [10, 12] alcohol intake [12] and radiation exposure [13].

Each factor carries a different power in terms of its ability to promote breast cancer. The strongest include genetic mutations, family history of breast cancer, age and previous history of an abnormal breast biopsy. It is in these groups of women that monitoring for breast cancer has been concentrated. Methods of surveillance include genetic counselling and yearly to three-yearly mammograms for detection of tumours in susceptible patients. This is labour-intensive often with a low pick up rate of tumours and with more knowledge of risk factors strongly implicated in the development the disease, recent research has been dedicated to identifying means to prevent breast cancer.

As each individual's risk of breast cancer varies, only some of the population will be at high enough risk to benefit from an intervention to reduce their chance of developing breast cancer. For this reason studies have investigated both the strength of each risk factor [14] and also how best to calculate each patient's probability of breast cancer. The most widely applicable model for risk assessment is the Gail model [15]. It was developed using prospective data of the above risk factors from 2,852 white women with breast cancer and 3,146 white women controls, all of whom underwent yearly breast cancer screening as part of the Breast Cancer Detection Demonstration Project. Unfortunately, only half of breast cancers occur in patients at with identifiable risk factors, so that limiting studies to this population would result in missing many who will develop breast cancers. With this in mind, more recent studies have investigated whether measurable biomarkers can help identify patients at increased risk and examples include mammographic breast density [16], serum hormone levels [17] and serum insulin growth factor-1 [18]. The methods for preventing breast cancer include reducing or antagonising estrogen using chemoprevention, anti-tumour agents and modifying lifestyle.

CHEMOPREVENTION

Clinical and experimental data have confirmed the link between estrogen and breast cancer. Trichopoulos and MacMahon showed that in women who underwent premenopausal oophorectomy, the relative risk of breast cancer fell from almost unity when this was performed at ≥ 50 to 0.36 when carried out at age <35 years [19]. Oophorectomy can lead to severe menopausal symptoms and so studies have examined the use of hormones to provide reversible antagonism with a lower profile of side effects.

Three aspects of estrogen modulation have been investigated. Firstly, gonadotrophin releasing hormone (GnRH) analogues have been used to antagonise the hypothalamic-pituitary pathway with add-back of estrogen. A second approach was selective estrogen receptor modulators (SERMs) which competitively bind to the estrogen receptor (ER). Tamoxifen has been the most widely used SERM because it is both effective with few side effects and has formed the basis of adjuvant hormonal therapy for many years [20]. More recently aromatase inhibitors to prevent peripheral generation of estrogen have been investigated.

In the first adjuvant tamoxifen trial there was a decrease of approximately 40% in the incidence of contralateral breast cancers [21]. Its use in the prevention of breast cancer was originally suggested in 1986 [22] following which, the Royal Marsden Hospital (RMH) began a pilot study to assess the effect of tamoxifen on the incidence of breast cancer in pre- and postmenopausal women with a family history of breast cancer. The pilot demonstrated that it was possible to recruit women to a chemoprevention trial with good compliance [23]. There followed a series of randomised, double blind, placebo-controlled trials that compared the effects of tamoxifen and later raloxifene against placebo on the incidence of breast cancer. The outline of the randomised prevention trials is given in Table 1.

NSABP

The largest of the trials was the National Surgical Adjuvant Breast and Bowel Project (NSABP) [24]. This enrolled 13,338 women aged ≥35 years into a trial comparing either 20mg tamoxifen or placebo over a five-year period. Participants had an increased risk of breast cancer as determined by the Gail model (1.66% risk or more), known previous history of LCIS or because they were older than 60 years of age. As well as breast cancer incidence the trial also examined side effects such as endometrial cancer, ischaemic heart disease events, fractures and vascular events. Potential participants were excluded if they had a history of deep vein thrombosis or pulmonary embolism. After a mean follow-up of 47 months there was a significant reduction in the incidence of both invasive and non-invasive breast cancer in the tamoxifen arm (124 cases v 244). The risk reduction was 49% for invasive and 50% for non-invasive cancer, but when analysed by subgroups, the risk reduction was greatest in women who were 60 years or older (55%) and those with previous LCIS (56%) or atypical duct hyperplasia (86%). When the tumour characteristics were examined the reduced incidence occurred only for ER+ tumours.

There was no significant difference in the incidence of ER- tumours nor in mortality rate for the 2 arms of the trial. Women in the tamoxifen group were at 2.53 times greater risk of developing endometrial cancer and 3 times more likely to suffer a pulmonary embolus, but both risks were significantly elevated only in post-menopausal women. Those taking tamoxifen were less likely to suffer fractures, particularly of the hip (49% risk reduction). There was no difference in the rate of ischaemic events but a greater incidence of hot flushes and vaginal discharge in the tamoxifen group. Once the trial results were published those participants taking placebo were allowed to start tamoxifen so that longer-term follow-up was not possible because of treatment contamination.

Table 1. Outline of randomized prevention trials

Trial	Number	Design	Follow-up	Ref
NSABP	13338	Tam 20mg v Plac	47 months	[24]
Royal Marsden	2471	Tam 20mg v Plac	70 months	[25]
IBIS-1	7152	Tam 20 mg v Plac	120 months	[32 33]
Italian	5408	Tam 20mg v Plac	46 months	[29 30]
MORE	7705	Ral 60mg v 120mg v Plac	96 months	[34]
CORE	4011	Ral 60mg v Plac	48 months	[35]
RUTH	10,101	Ral 60mg v Plac		[36]
STAR	19747	Tam 20m v Ral 60mg		[37]

Tam = Tamoxifen, Plac = Placebo, Ral = Raloxifene.

ROYAL MARSDEN HOSPITAL (RMH)

The Royal Marsden Hospital pilot study went on to recruit 2471 women with a family history of breast cancer into a trial with a median follow-up of 70 months [24]. In contrast to the NSABP trial there was no difference in the incidence of breast cancer in the tamoxifen and placebo groups [25]. There were significant differences between participants in the RMH trial compared with those in the NSABP study. Patients were younger (47 v 50-59), with a higher risk of developing breast cancer (96% v 76% had one first degree relative with breast cancer under the age of 50) and a larger proportion took HRT concomitantly with the tamoxifen (26% v <10%). The study authors reported that their participants had a >80% chance of holding a breast-cancer-predisposition gene, which could have impacted on the effectiveness of tamoxifen since the majority of tumours developing are ER negative. Furthermore, the concomitant use of HRT may have both reduced the efficacy of tamoxifen whilst elevating the risk of women in the placebo arm [26]. Follow up continued for up to 20 years (average of 13 years) and at this point, a significant reduction in breast cancer incidence was observed in the tamoxifen arm, predominantly in the post-treatment follow-up [27]. This difference was found only for ER+ve cancers.

ITALIAN TRIAL

The Italian study enrolled pre- and postmenopausal women, randomly assigned to either tamoxifen 20mg or placebo. To prevent development of endometrial cancer, all patients had undergone hysterectomy with or without oophorectomy. As oophorectomy reduces endogenous estrogen and is documented to reduce the development of invasive breast cancer, the consequence of this was that the risk of breast cancer within the study cohort was the same or even lower than the normal population [28]. In contrast to the NSABP study, analysis after 46 months [29] and 81 months [30] of follow-up revealed no difference in the incidence of breast cancer between the tamoxifen and placebo group. Subsequently, the authors stratified the study population using reproductive and hormonal characteristics into those at high risk or low risk of developing ER+ tumours. A retrospective analysis demonstrated that tamoxifen did reduce the incidence of breast cancer, but only in the high-risk subgroup of patients [31].

IBIS-I (INTERNATIONAL BREAST INCIDENCE STUDY)

IBIS-I recruited 7152 pre- and postmenopausal women with a family history of breast cancer and participants took either tamoxifen 20mg or placebo for five years. The primary outcome measured was the incidence of invasive and non-invasive breast cancer, secondary endpoints included the incidence of endometrial cancer, thromboembolic events and cardiovascular events. As in the NSABP trial, tamoxifen was found to reduce the incidence of both invasive breast cancer (25%) and non-invasive breast cancer (69%). All the risk reduction related to ER+ tumours: there was no reduction in ER- tumours [32]. Patients receiving tamoxifen suffered a greater rate of endometrial cancer; all women affected were postmenopausal, all but one were stage 1, low or intermediate grade adenocarcinoma and excess was non-significant. Other complications noted included a significant increase in the rate of thromboembolic events, vasomotor symptoms such as hot flushes and gynaecological symptoms such as abnormal bleeding. Long-term results from the study were released after 10 years of follow-up [33]. They demonstrated that the protective effect of tamoxifen lasted beyond the 5 years of treatment; the reduction between 0-5 years was 34% whilst between 5-10 years it was 22%. Furthermore, the percentage reduction of ER+ tumours was greater during the follow-up period than the treatment period (43% v 27%). There was no reduction in ER- tumours. These results suggest that the effects of tamoxifen accumulate during treatment giving further benefit beyond cessation of treatment. In contrast, the increased risk of endometrial cancers, thromboembolic events and cardiovascular events seen with tamoxifen was limited to the treatment period and not seen following its cessation.

MORE

Raloxifene is a selective estrogen receptor modulator that was developed for use in post-menopausal women with osteoporosis. The benefit of this is that it was as a common problem and so it could be of value to a larger proportion of women; 54% of breast cancers occur in women with a Gail evaluated risk of less than 1.67% - the cut off for the tamoxifen trials listed above. The disadvantage however was that all the trials involving raloxifene have limited participation to post-menopausal women.

The Multiple Outcomes of Raloxifene Evaluation (MORE) trial recruited 7705 postmenopausal women with evidence of osteoporosis to take 60mg raloxifene, 120mg raloxifene or placebo over a 40-month period. The primary endpoints included the incidence of breast cancer, endometrial thickness, deep vein thrombosis and pulmonary embolus (PE). There was a 76% decrease in all breast tumours; specifically 90% of ER+ tumours. It was calculated that 126 patients would need to be treated to prevent one case of breast cancer [34]. There was a similar increase in thromboembolic events as seen with tamoxifen but in contrast, raloxifene did not cause endometrial stimulation or carcinoma.

The drug was well tolerated; it was not associated with vaginal bleeding or breast pain, the main side effect being a high incidence of hot flushes.

CORE

Continuing Outcomes Relevant to Evista® is the follow-up trial from MORE. Patients, who were treated for more than 4 years whilst on the MORE trial were invited to participate in a double-blind placebo controlled study comparing raloxifene 60mg or placebo as randomised in the MORE trial. 4011 women were enrolled and completed a further 4 years of medication before analysis was performed. The trial showed a continuing effect of raloxifene in reducing the incidence of ER positive breast cancers (66% for the four years of the CORE trial, 76% for the 8 years of therapy). There was no difference identified in the rate of ER negative breast cancer between the raloxifene and placebo groups. After 8 years of therapy, there was no significant difference in adverse events between raloxifene and placebo groups in terms of vaginal bleeding, endometrial hyperplasia, endometrial cancer, risk of thromboembolic disease and breast pain. A statistical difference was noted in the reporting of leg cramps and hot flushes in the Raloxifene group after 8 years of therapy [35].

RUTH

The Raloxifene Use for The Heart (RUTH) trial also followed on from the MORE trial. It recruited 10,101 postmenopausal women with an increased risk of cardiovascular disease who were randomised to 60mg raloxifene or placebo for a period of 5 years. Primary outcomes measured included coronary events and invasive breast carcinoma. Despite evidence that raloxifene lowers levels of LDL cholesterol in this and other studies, analysis revealed no differences in the incidence of fatal and non-fatal myocardial infarction or hospitalisation from acute coronary syndrome between the raloxifene and placebo groups. However, with regards to the effect of raloxifene on the incidence of invasive breast cancer, there was a 55% reduction in ER+ cancers and no risk reduction for ER- tumours [36].

STAR

This was the second randomised, double blind prevention trial conducted by the National Surgical Adjuvant Breast and Bowel Project that directly compared tamoxifen and raloxifene. 19,747 postmenopausal women with a history of LCIS or breast cancer risk of over 1.66% (as estimated using the Gail method) were randomised to 5 years of either 20mg tamoxifen or 60mg raloxifene. There was no significant difference in the rates of invasive breast cancer between each group and a non-statistically significant rise in the rate of non-invasive breast cancer in the raloxifene group (80 v 57). In terms of adverse events; there was a trend for reduced incidence of endometrial cancer in the raloxifene group (23 v 36), and significant reductions in the rate of endometrial hyperplasia and hysterectomies performed. In addition, there was a 30% decrease in the rate of deep vein thrombosis and pulmonary embolism in the raloxifene group. No statistical difference was observed in the rate of other malignancies, ischaemic heart disease events, transient ischaemic attacks, fractures and deaths [37].

FURTHER AREAS TO BE INVESTIGATED

There is strong evidence for the use of tamoxifen and raloxifene in the prevention of breast cancer, and since raloxifene is associated with significantly fewer side effects in postmenopausal women it would be the drug of choice. However, its efficacy in pre-menopausal women has yet to be studied and it may be that its benefit in this group of women is not as strong as tamoxifen. Similarly, the adverse effects of tamoxifen appear to primarily affect postmenopausal women – suggesting that the risk/benefit ratio would be better in pre-menopausal women – allowing it to be used in this subset of the population. Nevertheless, its efficacy in this group has yet to be formally examined. It may be that as younger women are less likely to develop ER positive tumours and as such tamoxifen would not confer enough benefit to them. A Canadian group have used the findings of the BCPT trial and performed a statistical analysis to determine whether the normal population would benefit from tamoxifen based on the relative preventative benefit and potential detrimental adverse effects; their findings suggest that the risk/benefit ratio should limit tamoxifen use to those with a lifetime risk of >3.32%, which is much higher than the >1.66% for which it is currently approved [38]. Furthermore, when patients with a high risk of breast cancer are given the information of the potential benefits and risks associated with tamoxifen, the majority decline to take it based on fears of the potential adverse effects [39]. Additionally, tamoxifen and raloxifene do not protect against cardiovascular disease or osteoporosis to the same extent as hormonal replacement therapy – diseases that also present significant risk of morbidity in postmenopausal women, and concurrent use of HRT with tamoxifen could probably cancel its preventative effect.

In addition, there needs to be further assessment on the role of other estrogen derivatives or estrogen antagonism in breast cancer prevention. Aromatase inhibitors prevent the peripheral production of estrogens that serves as the major source of estrogen in postmenopausal women. It is already in use as an adjuvant therapy in post-menopausal women and its superiority over tamoxifen in reducing contralateral breast cancer was demonstrated in the Arimidex versus Tamoxifen Alone or in Combination (ATAC) trial [40]. Not only did anastrozole (Arimidex) reduce the incidence of contralateral breast cancers more than tamoxifen, but also with fewer reports of vaginal bleeding, thromboembolic events and endometrial cancer. Its main side effect is an increase in fractures and musculoskeletal symptoms. The IBIS group is currently examining the protective effects of anastrozole and exemestane in post-menopausal women as part of their IBIS-II trial whilst the National Cancer Institute of Canada's Clinical Trial Group (NCIC CTG) are studying its effectiveness when given in combination with cyclo-oxygenase (COX)-2 inhibitors. There are also studies into the role of gonadotrophin releasing hormone (GnRH) agonists, such as goserelin, which effectively produces a reversible oophorectomy. When used in combination with tamoxifen they have been shown to be effective as second-line endocrine therapy for pre-menopausal women with advanced breast cancer [41] and as effective as chemotherapy in the treatment of early hormone sensitive disease [42]. Goserelin has also been reported to reduce mammographic densities [43]. and there may be a preventative role for goserelin particularly in BRCA1 and BRCA2 patients [44] (discussed below).

Finally, there needs to be further assessment on the length of duration necessary for treatment. All the tamoxifen trials used 5 years worth of treatment and follow-up studies of both the RMH and IBIS-I trials have shown that the protective effects of tamoxifen outlast its treatment. However, extended treatment with raloxifene has been studied in the MORE and CORE trials which have shown that raloxifene continues to have a protective effect, albeit less than during the first four years of treatment – suggesting that unlike tamoxifen, there is no cumulative effect.

STRATEGIES IN PATIENTS CARRYING BRCA1/BRCA2 MUTATIONS

The breast cancer susceptibility genes BRCA1 and BRCA2 were identified, on the long arms of chromosomes 17 and 13 respectively, just over a decade ago. Mutations in these genes are thought to interact with p53 resulting in cell cycle dysfunction and failure to repair DNA damage [45]. They occur most commonly among Ashkenazi Jews at a rate of 2.5% and within their breast cancer population between 15 and 25% [46]. In the British population approximately 7% of breast cancers develop in patients with inherited mutations in BRCA1 or 2 [47].

These mutations predispose individuals to both breast and ovarian cancer from a young age. The lifetime risk of developing breast cancer can be as high as 80% [48] it being determined by both the penetration of the gene as well as age, family history of breast cancer and environmental factors such as age of menarche [49, 50]. The breast neoplasms developing in these patients are larger, of a higher grade and with a higher rate of ER receptor negativity [51]. Scandinavian studies show a strong correlation with negativity in BRCA1 carriers [52] but little association in BRCA2 carriers [53].

Prevention strategies for gene carriers include prophylactic mastectomy, oophorectomy, chemoprevention and oophorectomy with chemoprevention. The success of such approaches is difficult to analyse prospectively as BRCA1 and 2 carriers represent such a small population of patients who develop breast cancer and those in genetic testing programmes often already have been diagnosed with breast cancer. Of the limited studies available, with small patient numbers, most involve retrospective or observational studies, assessing a mixture of primary and secondary/contralateral disease [54]. The results indicate a potential benefit of 95% with prophylactic mastectomy [55], 50% with prophylactic oophorectomy [56], 63% with tamoxifen in BRCA2 carriers only and 84% with combined tamoxifen and oophorectomy (assessment of secondary contralateral breast cancer) [57]. There remains some confusion about the benefit of estrogen antagonism in BRCA1 carriers – patients with this mutation develop less ER positive tumours and studies investigating the potential benefit of tamoxifen suggest that estrogen antagonism confers little benefit [58]. However, this is in direct contrast to the finding that oophorectomy confers significant benefit – perhaps there is another variant of estrogen or estrogen receptor playing a role that is as yet unidentified?

ANTI-TUMOUR AGENTS

These include natural or synthetic agents that reverse or inhibit carcinogenesis. Studies have been performed to assess the benefit of vitamin A, vitamin E, selenium, gene/biological therapy and cyclo-oxygenase (COX)-2 inhibitors. Vitamin A analogues, retinoids, are natural antitumour agent and studies have documented their ability to interfere with the process of carcinogenesis [59]. A randomised trial of the benefit of 5 years therapy with Fenretinide in patients with previous breast cancer showed no effect on prevention of secondary cancer compared to placebo [60]. Longer follow-up did however show an effect in pre-menopausal women, in whom there was a significant risk reduction that increased with age and persisted beyond the treatment phase [61].

Vitamin E analogues such as α-Tocopherol are being investigated, as they are known to inhibit proliferation of tumour cells and induce apoptosis [62]. A study investigating the effects of dietary vitamins through the daily intake of fruits and vegetables in 83,234 women showed a reduction in risk of breast cancer in pre-menopausal women [63].

Selenium derivatives have also been found to have antitumour activity and studies suggest that it acts through active methylated metabolites formed in the body. Using a rat model of breast cancer an 86% reduction in risk was found after administration of Allylselenocysteine, a selenium compound, when compared with no treatment [64].

Gene therapy is based upon the idea of immunomodulation – activating the host immune system to fight tumours through mechanisms such as; introducing genes for cytokines into cancer cells to stimulate a cytotoxic response against the tumour [65] and directly introducing anti-tumour natural killer cells into the host [66]. This exciting concept has begun to develop with the discovery of recombinant DNA technology, however it is still far from therapeutic use. There are still multiple issues about how gene therapy is best delivered and the potential adverse effects of using viral agents or vaccines. In principle, it presents an ideal therapy by allowing a 'natural' treatment without potential side effects of surgery and chemotherapy.

COX-2 inhibitors were investigated as an over-expression of COX-2 is associated with the invasive capacity of aggressive tumours [67]. Cell studies assessing COX-2 expression in breast cancer, vascularisation and response to COX-2 inhibitors reveal that high levels of COX-2 are associated with a form of angiogenesis different to that seen in normal endothelial derived vasculature, which is reversed with the use of inhibitors. The hypothesis follows that COX-2 facilitates carcinogenesis by allowing this new type of vasculature to form in hypoxic or necrotic areas of breast cancer and that COX-2 inhibitors could therefore hinder carcinogenesis by preventing this vascular channel formation [68]. COX-2 has also been linked with aromatase induction [69] and growth of ER negative cell lines [70]. Rat mammary studies with the COX-2 inhibitor celecoxib, show a dose-dependant reduction in both the incidence and aggressive nature of tumours that increases with the addition of an aromatase inhibitor [71]. This synergistic relationship has prompted the National Cancer Institute of Canada's Clinical Trial Group NCIC CTG to begin a randomised trial of postmenopausal women with breast cancer to anastrozole versus exemestane for 5 years with or without celecoxib for 3 years. They are also launching a randomised phase III trial to assess the possible role of exemestane with or without celecoxib versus placebo in the prevention of breast cancer in postmenopausal women.

LIFESTYLE CHANGES

There is some work that suggests diet and exercise can reduce breast cancer risk [72]. Retrospective studies of athletes show a decrease incidence in the rate of breast and other cancers as well as adult-onset diabetes [73]. Regulation of diet, exercise and body mass index could act through reducing the circulating serum levels of estrogen [74] and sustaining a lean body [75]. It is unfortunate that many individuals would rather take a daily tablet than alter their lifestyle so that the applicability of these approaches remains questionable.

The major impediments to effective prevention of breast cancer are the large gaps in our knowledge of the aetiology of the disease: endocrine approaches will reduce the incidence of ER+ve cancer but different regimens are needed to inhibit the evolution of the more aggressive ER-ve variant. Once this has happened we will be able to look forward to the disappearance of this major killer of middle-aged women.

REFERENCES

[1]   Smigal C, Jemal A, Ward E, Cokkinides V, Smith R, Howe HL Thun M. Trends in breast cancer by race and ethnicity: update 2006. *CA: Cancer J.* 2006;56(3):168-183.

[2]   Easton DF, Bishop DT, Ford D, et al. Breast and ovarian cancer incidence in BRCA1-mutation carriers. *Am. J. Hum. Gen.* 1995;56:265-271.

[3]   Ries LAG, Eisner M, Kosary Cl, et al. SEER Cancer Statistics Review, 1973-1997. *NCI.* NIH publication. No. 00-2789. Bethesda, MD, 2000.

[4]   Brinton LA, Schaiere C, Hoover RN, et al. Menstrual factors and risk of breast cancer. *Cancer Invest.* 1988;249:145-154.

[5]   Brinton LA, Hoover R and Fraumeni JF Jr. Reproductive factors in the aetiology of breast cancer. *Br. J. Cancer* 1983;47:757-762.

[6]   Colditz GA, Stampfer MJ, Willet WC, et al. Prospective study of estrogen replacement therapy on the risk of breast cancer in postmenopausal women. *JAMA* 1990;265:1985-1990.

[7]   Nelso HD, Humphrey LL, Nygren P, et al. Postmenopausal hormone replacement therapy: scientific review. *JAMA* 2002;288:872-881.

[8]   Tretli S. Height and weight in relation to breast cancer morbidity and mortality. A prospective study of 570,000 women in Norway. *Int. J. Cancer* 1989;44:23-30.

[9]   Pharoah PDP, Day NE, Duffy S, et al. Family history and the risk of breast cancer: a systematic review and meta-analysis. *Int. J. Cancer* 1997;71:800-809.

[10]   Stybo Tm and Wood WD. The management of ductal and lobular breast cancer. *Surg. Oncol.* 1999;8:67-75.

[11]   Dupont WD, Park FF, Hartmann WH, et al. Breast cancer risk associated with proliferative breast disease and atypical hyperplasia. *Cancer* 1993;71:1258-1265.

[12]   Ellison RC, Zhang Y, McLennan CE, et al. Exploring the relation of alcohol consumption to risk of breast cancer. *Am. J. Epidemiol.* 2001;154:740-747.

[13]   Clemons S, Loijens L, Goss P. Breast cancer risk following irradiation for Hodgkin's disease. *Cancer Treat Rev.* 2000;26:291-302.

[14]   Singletary SE. Rating the risk factors for breast cancer. *Ann Surg* 2003;237(4):474-482.

[15] Gail MH, Brinton LA, Byar DP, et al. Projecting individualized probabilities of developing breast cancer for white females who are being examined annually. *J Natl. Cancer Inst.* 1989;81:1879-1886.

[16] Boyd NF, Martin LJ, Stone J, et al. Mammographic densities as a marker of human breast cancer risk and their use in chemoprevention. *Curr. Oncol. Rep.* 2001;3(4):314-321.

[17] Cauley JA, Lucas FL, Kuller LH, et al. Elevated serum estradiol and testosterone concentrations are associated with a high risk of breast cancer. *Ann. Int. Med.* 1999;130:270-277.

[18] Hankinson SE, Willet WC, Colditz GA, et al. Circulating concentrations of insulin-like growth factor-1 and the risk of breast cancer. *Lancet* 1998;9:1393-1396.

[19] Trichopoulos D, and MacMahon B. Menopause and breast cancer risk. *J. Natl. Cancer Inst.* (1972) 48 : 605-13.

[20] Nolvadex Adjuvant Trial Organization. Controlled trial of tamoxifen a single adjuvant in management of early breast cancer – analysis at six years by Nolvadex Adjuvant Trial Organization. *Lancet* 1985;1:836-839.

[21] Fornander T, Cedermark B, Mattson A, et al. Adjuvant tamoxifen in early breast cancer. Occurrence of new Primary cancers. *Lancet* 1989;ii:1070-1073.

[22] Cuzick J, Wang DY and Bulbrook RD. The prevention of breast cancer. *Lancet* 1986;i:83-86.

[23] Powles T, Hardy J, Ashely S, et al. A pilot trial to evaluate the acute toxicity and feasibility of tamoxifen for prevention of breast cancer. *Br. J. Cancer* 1989;60:126-131.

[24] Fisher B, Costantino JP, Wickerman DL, et al. Tamoxifen for Prevention of Breast Cancer: Report of the National Surgical Adjuvant Breast and Bowel Profect P-1 Study. *J. Natl. Cancer Inst.* 1998;90(18):1371-88

[25] Powles T, Eeles R, Ashley S, et al. Interim analysis of the incidence of breast cancer in the Royal Marsden Hospital tamoxifen randomized chemoprevention trial. *Lancet* 1998;352:98-101.

[26] The Collaborative Group on Hormonal Factors in Breast Cancer. Breast cancer and hormone replacement therapy: collaborative reanalysis of data from 51 epidemiological studies of 52,705 women with breast cancer and 108,411 women without breast cancer. *Lancet* 1997; 350: 1047-59.

[27] Powles TJ, Ashley S, Tidy A, et al. Twenty-year follow-up of the Royal Marsden randomized, double-blinded tamoxifen breast cancer prevention trial. *J. Natl. Cancer Inst.* 2007;99(4):283-90.

[28] Kelsey JL, Gammon MD, John EM. Reproductive factors and breast cancer. *Epidemiol Rev.* 1993;15:36-47.

[29] Veronesi U, Maisonneuve P, Coast A, et al. Prevention of breast cancer with tamoxifen: preliminary findings from the Italian randomized trial among hysterectomised women. *Lancet* 1998;352:93-7.

[30] Veronesi U, Maisonneuve P, Sacchini V, et al. The Italian Tamoxifen Study Group. Tamoxifen for breast cancer among hysterectomised women. *Lancet* 2002;359:1122-4.

[31] Vogel V and Lo S. Preventing Hormone-Dependent Breast Cancer in High-Risk Women. *J. Natl. Cancer Inst* 2003;95(2):91-93.

[32] IBIS investigators. First results from the International Breast Cancer Intervention Study (IBIS-I): a randomized prevention trial. *Lancet* 2002;360:817-824.

[33] Cuzick J, Forbes JF, Sestak I, et al. Long-term results of tamoxifen prophylaxis for breast cancer – 96 month follow-up of the randomized IBIS-I study. *J. Natl. Cancer Inst.* 2007;99:258-260.

[34] Cummings SR, Eckert S, Krueger KA et al. The Effect of Raloxifene on Risk Breast Cancer in Postmenopausal Women. *JAMA* 1999;281(23):2189-97.

[35] Martino S, Cauley JA, Barrett-Connor E, et al. CORE Investigators. Continuing outcomes relevant to Evista: breast cancer incidence in postmenopausal osteoporotic women in a randomized trial of raloxifene. *J. Natl. Cancer Inst.* 2004;96(23):1751-61.

[36] Barrett-Connor E, Mosca L, Collins P, et al. Effects of Raloxifene on Cardiovascular Events and Breast Cancer in Postmenopausal Women. *N. Eng. J. Med.* 2006;355(2):125-137.

[37] Vogel VG, Costantino JP, Wickerman DL, et al. Effects of Tamoxifen vs Raloxifene on the Risk of Developing Invasive Breast Cancer and Other Disease Outcomes. The NSABP Study of Tamoxifen and Raloxifene (STAR) P-2 trial. *JAMA* 2006;295(23):2727-2741.

[38] Will BP, Nobrega KM, Berthelot J-M, et al. First do no harm: extending the debate on the provision of preventative tamoxifen. *Br. J. Cancer* 2001;85(9):1280-1288.

[39] Port ER, Montgomery LL, Heerdt AS and Borgen PI. Patient reluctance toward tamoxifen use for breast cancer primary prevention. *Ann. Surg. Oncol.* 2001;8(7):580-585.

[40] The ATAC Trialists' Group. Arimidex, Tamoxifen Alone or in Combination, Anastrozole alone or in combination with tamoxifen versus tamoxfien alone for adjuvant treatment of postmenopausal

women with early breast cancer: first results of the ATAC randomised trial. *Lancet* 2002;359(9324):2131-2139.

[41] Forward DP, Cheung KL, Jackson L and Robertson JFR. Clinical and endocrine data for goserelin plus anastrozole as second-line endocrine therapy for premenopausal advanced breast cancer. *Br. J. Cancer* 2004;90:590-594.

[42] Kauffman M, on behalf of the ZEBRA Trialists' Group. Zoladex™ (goserelin) versus CMF as adjuvant therapy in pre/perimenopausal, node-positive, early breast cancer: preliminary efficacy results from the ZEBRA study. *Breast* 2001;10(Suppl1):S30.

[43] Spicer DV, Ursin G, Parisky YR, et al. Changes in mammographic densities induced by a hormonal contraceptive designed to reduce breast cancer risk. *J Natl Cancer Inst* 1994;86(6):431-436.

[44] Wirk B. The role of ovarian ablation in the management of breast cancer. *Breast Jl* 2005;11(6):416-424.

[45] Phillips K-A, Nichol K, Ozcelik H, et al. Frequency of p53 mutations in breast carcinomas from Ashkenazi Jewish carriers of BRCA1 mutations. *J. Natl. Cancer Inst.* 1999;91: 469-73.

[46] Warner E, Foulkes W, Goodwin P, et al. Prevalence and penetrance of BRCA1 and BRCA2 gene mutations in unselected Ashkenazi Jewish women with breast cancer. *J. Natl. Cancer Inst.* 1999;91:1241-7.

[47] Claus EB, Schildkraut JM, Thompson WD and Risch NJ. The genetic attributable risk of breast and ovarian cancer. *Cancer* 1996;77:2318-2324.

[48] Arver B, Du Q, Chen J, Luo L and Lindblom A. Hereditary breast cancer: a review. *Sem. Cancer Biol.* 2000;10:271-288.

[49] Easton DF, Ford D and Bishop DT. Breast and ovarian cancer incidence in BRCA1-mutation carriers. Breast cancer link consortium. *Am. J. Hum. Gen.* 1995;56(1):265-271.

[50] Antoniou A, Pharoah PD, Narod S, et al. Average risks of breast and ovarian cancer associated with BRCA1 or BRCA2 mutations detected in case series unselected for family history: a combined analysis of 22 studies. *Am J Hum Gen* 2003;72:1117-30.

[51] Breast Cancer Link Consortium. Pathology of familial breast cancer: differences between breast cancers of BRCA1 or BRCA2 mutations and sporadic cases. *Lancet* 1997;349:1505-1510.

[52] Johannsson OT, Idvall I, Anderson C, et al. Tumour biological features of BRCA1-induced breast and ovarian cancer. *Eur. J. Cancer* 1997;33:362-371.

[53] Loman N, Johannsson O, Bendahl PO, et al. Steroid receptors in hereditary breast carcinomas associated with BRCA1 or BRCA2 mutations or unknown susceptible genes. *Cancer* 1998;83:310-319.

[54] Calderon-Margalit R and Paltiel O. Prevention of breast cancer in women who carry BRCA1 or BRCA2 mutations: a critical review of the literature. *Int. J. Cancer* 2204;112:357-364.

[55] Rebbeck TR, Friebel T, Lynch HT, et al. Bilateral prophylactic mastectomy reduces breast cancer risk in BRCA1 and BRCA2 mutation carriers: the PORSE Study Group. *J. Clin. Oncol.* 2004;22:1055-1062.

[56] Rebbeck TR, Lynch HT, Neuhausen SL, et al. The Prevention and Observation of Surgical End Points Study Group: prophylactic oophorectomy in carriers of BRCA1 or BRCA2 mutations. *N. Engl. J. Med.* 2002;346:1616-1622.

[57] Narod SA, Brunet JS, Gharirian P, et al. Tamoxifen and risk of contralateral breast cancer in BRCA1 and BRCA2 mutation carriers: a case-control study. Hereditary Breast Cancer Clinical Study Group. *Lancet* 2000;356:1876-1881.

[58] Duffy SW and Nixon RM. Estimates of the likely prophylactic effect of tamoxifen in women with high risk BRCA1 and BRCA2 mutations. *Br. J. Cancer* 2002;86:218-221.

[59] Lippman SM, Lee JJ, Sabichi AL. Cancer chemoprevention: progress and promise. *J. Natl. Cancer Inst.* 1998;90:1514-1528.

[60] Veronesi U, De Palo G, Marubini E, et al. Randomized trial of fenretinide to prevent second breast malignancy in women with early breast cancer. *J. Natl. Cancer Inst.* 1999;91(21):1847-1856.

[61] Veronesi U, Mariani L, Decensi A, et al. Fifteen-year results of a randomised phase III trial of fenretinide to prevent second breast cancer. *Ann. Oncol.* 2006;17:1065-1071.

[62] Neuzil J. Vitamin E succinate and cancer treatment: a vitamin E prototype for selective antitumour activity. *Br. J. Cancer* 2003;89:1822-1826.

[63] Zhang S, Hunter DJ, Forman MR, et al. Dietary carotenoids and vitamins A, C and E and risk of breast cancer. *J. Natl. Cancer Inst.* 1999;91:547-556.

[64] Clement IP, Zhu Z, Thompson HJ, Lisk D and Ganther HE. Chemoprevention of mammary cancer with Se-Allylselenocysteine and other selenoamino acids in the rat. *Anticancer Res.* 1999;19:2875-2880.

[65] Gutierrez AA, Lemoine NR and Sikora K. Gene therapy for cancer. *Lancet* 1992;339:715-721.

[66] Rosenberg SA. Immunotherapy and gene therapy of cancer. *Cancer Res (Suppl.)* 1991;51:5074s-5079s.

[67] Rozic JG, Chakraborty C and Lala PK. Cyclooxygenase inhibitors retard murine mammary tumor progression by reducing tumor cell migration, invasiveness and angiogenesis. *Int. J. Cancer.* 2001;93:497–506.

[68] Basu GD, Liang WS, Stephan DA, et al. A novel role for cyclooxygenase-2 in regulating vascular channel formation by human breast cancer cells *Breast Cancer Res.* 2006;8(6):R69.

[69] Howe LR, Subbaramaiah K, Brown AM and Dannenberg AJ. Cyclo-oxygenase-2: a target for the prevention and treatment of breast cancer. *Endocr Rel Cancer* 2001;8(2):97-114.

[70] Arun B, Zhang H, Mirza GN, et al. Growth inhibition of breast cancer cells by celecoxib. *Breast Cancer Res. Treat* 2001;69(3):234.

[71] Pesenti E, Masferrer JL and di Salle E. Effect of exemestane and celecoxib alone or in combination on DMBA-induced mammary carcinoma in rats. *Breast Cancer Res Treat* 2001;69(3):288.

[72] Verloop J, Rookus MA, van der Kooy K and Leeuwen FE. Physical activity and breast cancer risk in women aged 20-5 years. *J Natl Cancer Inst* 2000;92(2):128-135.

[73] Fintor L. Exercise and breast cancer risk: lacking consensus. *J. Natl. Cancer Inst.* 1999;91(10):825-827.

[74] Broocks A, Pirke KM, Schweiger U, et al. Cyclic ovarian function in recreational athletes. *J. Appl. Physiol.* 1990;68:2083-2086.

[75] Carpenter CL, Ross RK, Paganini-Hill A and Bernstein L. Lifetime exercise activity and breast cancer risk among post-menopausal women. *Br. J. Cancer* 1999;80(11):1852-1858.

In: Breast Cancer Screening and Prevention   ISBN 978-1-61209-288-1
Editor: Jonathan D. Pegg   © 2011 Nova Science Publishers, Inc.

Chapter 2

HEALTH BELIEFS AND BREAST CANCER SCREENING: APPLYING THE STAGE-OF-CHANGE MODELS

Mª José Galdón, Estrella Durá*,
Yolanda Andreu, Silvia Queipo and Elena Ibáñez
Department of Personality, Assessment and Psychological Treatments,
University of Valencia, Valencia, Spain

Reviewed by
Etzel Cardeña
Departament of Psychology, University of Lund, Lund (Sweden)
Lea Baider
Department of Radiation and Clinical Oncology, Sharett Institute of
Oncology, Hadassah University Hospital. Jerusalem (Israel)

---

* Corresponding Author: Estrella Durá. Departamento de Personalidad. Facultad de Psicología. Avnda. Blasco Ibañez, Nº 21, 46010 Valencia (Spain). Tel.: + 34 96 386 4476. Fax: + 34 96 386 4669. E-mail address: estrella.dura@uv.es

ABSTRACT

This research analyzes the beliefs and attitudes towards breast cancer and mammography –using the sociocognitive postulated by the health beliefs models- associated with different stages of mammography adoption. A cross-sectional design were used. The sample was consisting of Spanish women (N= 151), aged 47-70 years. They were evaluated by the same questionnaire, which measured two types of variables: (i) Socio-cognitive: perceived severity of breast cancer, perceived susceptibility to breast cancer, general health motivation, benefits and barriers perceived to mammography, social pressure, perceived control on this preventive behaviour and the degree of information about breast cancer screening; and (ii) Stage of mammography adoption: Precontemplation, Contemplation, Action, Action-Maintenance and Relapse. All the cognitive variables, except the perceived susceptibility to breast cancer, have significant differences depending on the stage of mammography adoption. According to the stages of adoption, the women differ as for their beliefs towards mammography screening and breast cancer, differ also in the control and social pressure that they perceive to undergo mammograms, and in the degree of information that they have about breast cancer screening mammography. The results of this research may inform interventions to increase mammography use.

1. INTRODUCTION

The mammogram is the most widely known technique for early breast cancer detection (Humphrey, Helfand, Chand and Wolf, 2002; Kerlikowke, Grady, Rubin, Sandrock and Ernster 1995; Primic-Zakelj, 1999; Rippon, 1994). Research shows that periodic mammography screening reduces the mortality rate caused by breast cancer among women aged between 40 and 47 (Humphrey et al., 2002). This effect the screening has on breast cancer mortality is persistent throughout long-term follow-ups and is age dependent, obtaining better results on women over fifty (Deck and Kakuma, 2005; Nystrom et al., 2002). Although some authors have questioned the utility of breast cancer screening (Gotzsche and Olsen, 2000; Olsen and Gotzsche, 2001), and there is still controversy regarding the age of initiation (Miller, Baines and To, 2002; Ringash, 2001; Sox, 2002), there is consensus as to the recommendation (grade B) of screening: every 1 or 2 years for early breast cancer detection in women aged 40 and over (Agency for Healthcare Research and Quality, 2002).

Furthermore, it is necessary to take into account that the success of any early detection program does not solely depend on the clinical effectiveness of the screening technique used—the mammogram in this case—but also on the participation by the targeted population. Without high participation rates, no screening program will meet necessary and essential requirements to achieve its goals (Marteau, 1994). Even though women's participation standards in screening programs have increased substantially in recent years -mainly due to their implementation by organizations and public institutions- they are still, on some occasions, lower than desired (George, 2000; Meystre-Agustoni, Dubois-Arber, Landstheer and Paccaud, 1998; Pelfrene, Bleyen and Backer, 1998). For this reason, studies of psychosocial factors associated with the participation in mammography screening constitute a primary objective regarding the early detection of breast cancer.

The Health Belief Model and the Theory of Reasoned Action have traditionally received more attention on behalf of psychologists when it comes to understanding the factors that influence mammography attendance.

The Health Belief Model (HBM) (Rosenstock, 1966) contains three main elements. First of all, the perceived threat of the illness determined by the individual's perceptions of *susceptibility* to it, and by the perceived *severity* of the consequences of contracting it. Secondly, the individual's assessment of the *benefits* of adopting preventative behavior balanced against *barriers* that may emerge such as the economic cost, or psychological effects, or others of a different nature. The perceived threat would determine the degree of the individual's psychological motivation or preparation to perform any preventative action; the specific action undertaken would be subject to the consideration of the perceived benefits and barriers of each of the considered actions. Thirdly, the necessary motivation for the individual to perform the behavior would be constituted by the presence of a *cue to action*, either internal (i.e., symptoms) or external (i.e., seeing how a close relative dies because of the illness). In recent years, however, some of the HBM's authors (Rosenstock, Strecher and Becker, 1988; Rosenstock, 1990) have suggested expanding the model to include other variables such as *general health motivation* or value that the person gives to his/her health (Becker, 1974); the degree by which the individual's health is perceived as being under one's own control or beyond it -*health locus of health control*- Wallston, 1992) and the expectation of self-efficacy or the individual's belief in one's own skill to perform the preventative behavior correctly (Bandura, 1977, 1997).

The Theory of Reasoned Action (TRA) (Ajzen and Fishbein, 1980) proposes that the immediate antecedent of the behavior is the *intention* to perform it; this is, at the same time, a function of two factors: (i) the individual's *attitudes* towards the behavior -assessed as the product of the person's beliefs about the consequences of the behavior and his/her assessment of these consequences-; and (ii) the *subjective norms* – a person's beliefs about whether significant other think he or she should engage in the behavior (social pressure) and one's motivation to respond to these perceived requirements. Recently, Ajzen (1998, 1991) has suggested the addition of another variable: the *perceived behavioral control*. According to the author, the perceived capacity of an individual to exercise voluntary control on the behavior in question will not just influence his/her intention to perform it, but also its true execution. The new version of the theory that includes the perceived behavioral control has been renamed as Theory of Planned Behavior (TPB).

Both models acknowledge that other variables such as sociodemographics, personality characteristics or the degree of information (generically known as structural variables) can have an influence on the decision to adopt a health behavior, but always indirectly, through its influence on the basic sociocognitive dimensions proposed by the model.

When these theoretical models have been applied to the study of the mammography behavior, the results obtained have generally shown the existence of significant relations between the examined variables in these models and preventative behavior, although the explained variance percentages are moderate and, in general, lower than expected according to the theoretical assumptions (for revision, see Durá, Andreu and Galdón, 2001; Galdón, Durá, Andreu, Tuells and Ibáñez, 2003). Moreover, several authors have pointed out some constraints in these theoretical frameworks, mainly for being considered static models which are interested exclusively in people's motivations to perform health behaviors, but without approaching the problem of how intentions become actions and/or how processes of changes in health behaviors are produced (Conner and Norman, 2001; Sheeran and Abraham, 1996).

Regarding this line of argument, a series of recent research studies on screening behavior are based on the assumption that the adoption of a health behavior, such as periodical screening, should not be conceptualized as a dichotomy of meeting a given criterion or not, but as a process. The theoretical framework of this new approach is made up of the *stages-of-change models* that have successfully been applied to the study of the abandonment of addictive behaviors such as alcoholism or tobacco (DiClemente and Hughes, 1990; Prochaska and DiClemente, 1983; Weinstein, 1988) and that have been gaining ground in the research on health behaviors, including breast cancer screening.

Among the stage models, the Transtheoretical Model (TTM) (Prochaska and DiClemente, 1982) has been the one that has focused its attention on the study of screening behavior. This model conceptualizes behavior change as a process, postulating that individuals move through a series of *stages* that are progressively more implicated in the adoption of a health behavior or its abandonment. Thus, the model facilitates a classification outline of the individuals in the case that they have not even considered the behavior in question (precontemplation); that they are considering it but they have not taken any action (contemplation); that they are in a consolidated phase of the behavioral change (maintenance); or, even in the case that they have begun the action at any time but they have not maintained it (relapse). Apart from these stages, the model postulates other elements that are responsible for the progression, maintenance and/or abandonment of the health behavior: the *processes-of-change* (concealed and/or manifest activities that individuals perform when they try to modify a health behavior); and the *decisional balance* or pros and cons of the behavior in question (the perceived positive and negative aspects of such behavior). These concepts explain the movements from one stage to another and they are empirically associated to them (Prochaska and DiClemente, 1983).

The TTM has been applied either using its own concepts exclusively: stages, decisional balance, and processes of change (Chamot, Charvet and Perneger, 2001; Clark et al., 1998; Rakowski et al., 1992, Rakowski, Fulton, and Feldman, 1993; Rakowski et al., 1996, 1997a, 1997b; Rimer et al., 1996; Stoddard et al., 1998) or in combination with the HBM -comparing the variables of the benefits and barriers of this model with the pros and cons of the transtheoretical model (Brenes and Skinner, 1999; Champion, 1994; Champion and Skinner, 2003; Champion and Springston, 1999; Skinner, Champion, Gonin and Hanna, 1997; Skinner, Kreuter, Kobrin and Strecher, 1998a). In both cases, the results show significant differences in womens' perceptions of the mammography depending on their current stage of adoption. In addition, recent research on the transtheoretical model has shown that the interventions specifically designed according to the current stage of mammography adoption, significantly increase the adherence to screening controls (Champion et al., 2003; Clark et al., 2002; Crane et al., 2000; Lipkus,

Rimer, Halabi, and Strigo, 2000; Rakoswki et al., 1998; Skinner, Strecher and Hospers, 1994; Rimer et al., 2001;).

Precisely with the main objective of directing the programs towards increasing women's screening attendance, this research analyzes the beliefs and attitudes towards breast cancer and mammography -using the sociocognitive variables postulated by the health belief models- associated with different stages of mammography adoption.

2. METHOD

2.1. Design

A cross-sectional design was used. Five groups of women were established according to their stage of mammography adoption.

2.2. Sample

Two exclusion criteria were considered for the selection of the sample: aged 70 and over, or under the age of 47; and their personal history of breast cancer The sample has been formed by a group of a total of 151 women, with an mean age of 59 (SD= 7.39). The majority of women who participated in the study had an elementary education at the most (69%) and only 14.6% had a higher education. The sample was subdivided into five groups of women according to their individual stage of mammography adoption.

2.3. Procedure

The sample was obtained from different women's associations (neighborhoods, housewives' associations, dance halls, etc...), as well as from particular and individual contacts. All the women in the sample lived in the city of Valencia (Spain) or in surrounding urban areas. The participation of women was voluntary and their answers were anonymous. All of them were given the same questionnaire. In some cases they were conducted in groups where instructions on how to fill in the questionnaire were duly given, and in other cases (the majority) questionnaires were conducted individually by a psychologist.

2.4. Variables and Instruments

Two types of variables have been assessed: the stage of mammography adoption and different sociocognitive variables in reference to beliefs and attitudes towards breast cancer and screening. The following instruments were used:

Scale for the stages of mammography adoption. This gathers information on the screening controls that were undergone by each of the women. This scale consists of 6 items, each one with different answer alternatives. Four of them were used to define the stages of mammography adoption and contain information about matters such as: if the subject has had a mammogram before and, if so, how often, how long has it been since the last mammogram, and from the last one to the previous one, and finally whether she plans to undergo screening within a maximum period of two years or not. These items were elaborated from the definitions of stages of adoption published in different studies related to the Transtheoretical Model and preventative breast cancer behaviors (Champion, 1994; Clark et al., 1998; Rakowski et al., 1993; Rakowski et al., 1997a, 1997b; Skinner et al., 1997; Skinner, Arfken and Sykes, 1998b). Two other items asked about the reasons and the place where the mammogram was performed, in this case, with the objective of excluding those women who had mammograms for reasons other than those related to breast cancer screening.

The stages of mammography adoption utilized in this research were determined from the following criteria:

Precontemplation: has never had a mammogram and does not plan to have one in the next two years.

Contemplation: has never had a mammogram, but intends to have one in the next two years.

Action: has had a mammogram in the last two years, but has not had any in the two previous years (that is to say, 4 years ago) and is planning to have another one in the next two years.

Action/Maintenance: had a mammogram two years ago, another one two years before and intends to have another one in the next two years.

Relapse: has had a previous mammogram, but not in the last two years, and intends to have one in the next two years; or had one previously in the last two years and does not intend to have any in the next two years.

Questionnaire regarding the degree of information about the techniques of early breast cancer detection. Composed of 9 items that quantify the degree of information about the techniques of breast cancer's secondary prevention. It has been elaborated from the instruments on the degree of information about breast cancer, published by Stillman (1977) and McCance, Mooney, Smith and Field (1990).

Scale about beliefs and attitudes towards breast cancer. The variables "perceived susceptibility" to breast cancer (5 items), "perceived severity" of the illness (7 items) and "general health motivation" (7 items) from the Health Belief Models are assessed by the questionnaire elaborated by Champion (1993). All the items were assessed with a 7-point Likert format (from "strongly disagree" to "strongly agree").

Scale of perceived consequences of the mammogram. From questionnaires by different authors (Champion, 1993; Montano and Taplin 1991; Rakowski et al., 1993, 1997; Skinner et al. 1997, 1998b; Stein, Fox, Murata and Morisky, 1992; Vaile, Calnan, Rutter and Wall, 1993), corresponding measures were taken for the "perceived benefits" –pros- and "perceived barriers" –cons- variables of the mammogram. The benefits subscale is made up of a total of 14 items and the barrier subscale is made up of 17. All of them are presented in a 7-point Likert format (from "strongly disagree" to "strongly agree").

Scale about perceived social pressure. From an adaptation of the questionnaires by Vaile et al. (1993) and from Montano and Taplin (1991), this variable proposed by the Theory of Reasoned Action is assessed. The scale is made up of 7 items with a 7-point Likert format (from "strongly disagree" to "strongly agree") that test the degree of pressure that the person perceives from significant others to have mammograms.

Perceived control scale. Two items were elaborated for the assessment of the "perceived control" variable, proposed by the Theory of Planned Behavior, also with a 7-point Likert format from "not at all" to "absolutely", which assess the degree of control that women perceive when they go to have mammograms.

The internal consistency of the assessment scales of the sociocognitive variables is generally satisfactory: "information" ($\alpha=.83$), "severity" ($\alpha=.73$), "susceptibility" ($\alpha=.87$), "general health motivation" ($\alpha=.76$), "benefits" ($\alpha=.90$), "barriers" ($\alpha=.89$), and "social pressure" ($\alpha=.83$). Only the "Perceived control" scale showed a low coefficient ($\alpha=0.50$); that is why in all analyses in which this variable was involved, analyses with the complete scale were carried out and with each of the two items that constitute it independently. Given that the results obtained do not differ according to how they were assessed, the analyses with the complete scale are shown exclusively.

2.5. Statistical Analyses

After subdividing the whole sample into five groups according to the stage of mammography adoption, a multivariate analysis of covariance (MANCOVA) was run with its corresponding *post hoc* tests for the study of the assessed sociocognitive variables, in order to analyze the existence of significant differences in these variables between the subgroups. Furthermore, and in order to analyze the specific beliefs associated with the stage of mammography adoption, we ran analyses of covariance (ANCOVAs) and the corresponding *post hoc* tests for the items of those variables in which this analysis could add qualitatively notable information beyond the one offered by the total score of the scale: "benefits", "barriers" and "information".

In the Mancova we check the homogeneity of covariance matrices by means of the Box's M test, and given that it proved to be significant, we proceeded to the use of the contrast statistics, Traza de Pillai, since it is a more robust test recommended in case of small samples or if the homogeneity of covariances is unreliable (Hair, Anderson, Tatham and Black, 1999). In the contrasting tests between subgroups we used the Bonferroni test because it adjusts the observed significance level when you perform multiple comparisons.

3. RESULTS

3.1. Differences between Stages in Sociocognitive Variables

Before analyzing the existence of differences in the sociocognitive variables among the different stages of the mammography adoption, it was decided to check if there were any differences between the stages at sociodemographic variables. In Table 1 mean age and percentages of education levels are shown for each stage. The analyses of the differences between stage groups showed statistically significant differences both for age (F= 5.31; p=.001) and education level (Chi squared=26.75; p=.008). For this reason, it was decided to control this effect on the possible differences between stages in sociocognitive variables, introducing them as covaried variables in future analyses.

Using sociocognitive variables as dependent variables; sociodemographic ones as covaried, and the stage as an independent variable, the Mancova showed the existence of significant effects of this last variable (Traza de Pillai: [27.101]=0.61; p=0.00). In Table 2, the mean and standard deviation in the sociocognitive variables of each stage group, along with the results of the F-test and the significance level are shown. Table 3 shows the results for post hoc test which reached statistical significance (p<.05).

Mancova's results (see Table 2) show that all the assessed sociocognitive variables, except *susceptibility*, establish statistically significant differences between the stages. Nevertheless, in the post hoc tests (see Table 3) the *severity* variable does not reach statistic significance in any of them, perhaps due to the small size of the sample in some subgroups. These post hoc tests indicate that a large majority of the differences are established between the precontemplation group (G1) vs. the action (G3) and action/maintenance (G4) groups. Given the means (Table 1), the precontemplation group vs. the other two groups significantly shows less *information* and less *general health motivation*; it perceives fewer *benefits* and more *barriers*; and shows less *control* over this technique; it also perceives significantly less *social pressure* particularly compared to the action group (G3). This precontemplation group (G1) also perceives (in a statistically significant way) fewer *benefits* of the mammogram screening in comparison with the contemplation (G2) and relapse (G5) groups.

Statistically significant differences are also visible between the relapse group (G5) and the action (G3) and action/maintenance (G4) groups. Significantly compared to the other two, the first one shows fewer *benefits* and less *information*; it also shows more *barriers* in comparison with G4. Finally, the contemplation group (G2), perceives significantly fewer *benefits* than the action group (G3).

3.2. Differences between Stages in the Perceived Benefits Items

Covariance analyses were run (ANCOVAs) for each item of the benefits variable. Table 4 shows means and standard deviations of each stage, along with the results of the F-test and the significance level. In Table 5, contrasts between the groups that reached statistical significance (p<.05) are shown.

The results (see Table 4) indicate that only one item does not establish significant differences between groups. Most of the differences (see Table 5) are established between the precontemplation group (G1) and the rest. Thus, given the means (Table 4), the women in this group believe, to a significantly lesser extent than all the rest, that the mammogram would enable an early diagnosis if they had breast cancer (item 2); it would confirm that everything is going well (item1) and nothing is wrong (item 5); and it would provide them with control over their health (item 14). Moreover, this precontemplation group (G1) obtains scores which are significantly lower than the action (G3) and action/maintenance (G4) groups in the other six benefits related to the peace of mind that this screening technique provides (items 9, 10, 11) and with the belief in its effectiveness to control the illness by means of an earlier treatment (items 4, 12, 13). Moreover, the precontemplation group (G1), vs. the action group (G3), is less likely to believe: a mammogram would detect abnormalities and non-cancerous lumps (item 3); it would detect cancer that could not have been found by means of breast self-examination (item 6); it would reduce the probability of death from breast cancer (item 8).

Table 1. Mean and percentages (%) in sociodemographic variables for each of the stage groups

STAGE	Mean age	% Percentages education level			
		None	Primary	Secondary	Higher
Precontemplation N =24	62.9	33.3	41.7	8.3	16.7
Contemplation N = 20	55.2	10.0	45.0	30.0	15.0
Action N = 29	61.3	17.2	55.2	20.7	6.9
Action-Maintenance N = 56	57.0	1.8	53.6	25.0	19.6
Relapse N = 22	59.9	0.0	68.2	22.7	9.1

Table 2. MANCOVA for the sociocognitive variables. Test F and significance level. Means and standard deviations from the variables in each of the groups

Variables	F	p	G1 N=24 X	SD	G2 N=20 X	SD	G3 N=29 X	SD	G4 N=56 X	SD	G5 N=22 X	SD
Severity	4.31	0.00	33.46	9.46	33.60	8.61	35.41	7.96	29.71	8.32	30.91	11.50
Susceptibility	0.90	0.50	13.67	8.34	13.45	7.87	12	6.58	13.14	7.30	12.46	7.74
HealthMotivation	4.06	0.00	20.25	5.39	22.80	4.80	25.83	3.33	24.38	4.82	22.14	6.68
Benefits	16.80	0.00	62.75	16.80	80.40	12.70	89.14	7.78	87.64	9.12	76.36	17.20
Barriers	5.42	0.00	70.58	22.74	54.60	18.17	52.38	16.42	49.05	25.45	68.27	22.39
Information	13.77	0.00	4.69	3.28	6.83	2.49	7.19	1.56	7.69	1.17	5.47	2.44
Social pressure	2.44	0.03	31.25	7.35	35.75	8.63	38.72	7.67	37.34	9.99	35.50	8.49
Perceived control	5.96	0.00	8.71	4.38	9.90	2.77	11.79	2.61	12.09	2.85	9.50	4.00

X = mean. SD= standard deviation. p= significance. Significant information is shaded.
G1= Precontemplation; G2= Contemplation; G3= Action; G4= Action-Maintenance; G5= Relapse.

Table 3. Post hoc tests between groups for sociocognitive variables that reached statistical significance (Bonferroni's test)

Variables	G1-G2	G1-G3	G1-G4	G1-G5	G2-G3	G3-G5	G4-G5
Severity							
Susceptibility							
Health Motivation		5.42***	3.64*				
Benefits	14.50**	25.75***	22.87***	12.67**	11.26*	13.08*	10.19**
Barriers		17.47*	17.66*				17.59*
Information		2.33***	2.23***			1.97**	1.88**
Social pressure		7.17*					
Perceived control		2.91**	2.72**				

Significance Levels: $* \leq 0.05$; $** \leq 0.01$; $*** \leq 0.001$.
G1= Precontemplation; G2= Contemplation; G3= Action; G4= Action-Maintenance; G5= Relapse.

Table 4. ANCOVAs for each of the items of the *benefits* variable. Test F and significance level. Means and standard deviations of the items in each of the groups

Benefits* Items	F	p	G1 N = 24 X	SD	G2 N = 20 X	SD	G3 N = 29 X	SD	G4 N = 56 X	SD	G5 N = 22 X	SD
Item 1	9.15	0.00	3.88	1.94	5.85	1.39	6.66	0.77	6.27	1.42	5.27	2.39
Item 2	6.09	0.00	5.13	1.33	6.50	0.83	6.66	0.94	6.54	1.11	6.27	1.61
Item 3	4.85	0.00	5.50	1.22	5.90	1.52	6.72	0.46	6.57	1.06	5.55	2.11
Item 4	5.63	0.00	5.13	1.45	6.10	0.85	6.72	0.59	6.55	1.16	6.18	1.71
Item 5	6.25	0.00	4.25	1.87	6.05	1.05	6.28	1.62	6.16	1.52	5.77	1.80
Item 6	6.34	0.00	5.21	1.29	5.95	1.47	6.52	1.21	6.71	0.91	6.23	1.27
Item 7	1.65	0.14	5.46	1.18	5.90	1.33	6.48	0.91	6.00	1.64	5.73	2.00
Item 8	3.47	0.00	3.00	2.00	4.95	1.99	5.04	2.26	4.91	2.40	4.09	2.67
Item 9	9.48	0.00	4.13	1.87	5.65	1.53	6.52	1.30	6.52	1.19	5.46	2.11
Item 10	4.38	0.00	3.79	1.79	5.20	1.61	5.66	2.09	5.84	1.85	4.96	2.06
Item 11	6.20	0.00	4.29	1.66	5.40	1.43	6.21	1.18	6.34	1.41	5.18	2.20
Item 12	4.00	0.00	4.58	1.50	5.60	1.23	6.41	1.05	5.91	1.92	5.14	1.96
Item 13	10.59	0.00	4.58	1.64	5.50	1.43	6.62	1.24	6.73	0.82	5.23	2.05
Item 14	14.07	0.00	3.83	1.93	5.85	1.27	6.65	0.61	6.59	1.06	5.32	2.12

X = media. SD= standard deviation. p= significance. The significant information is shaded. G1= Precontemplation; G2= Contemplation; G3= Action; G4= Action-Maintenance; G5= Relapse. * In Appendix 1 the formulation of the items is shown.

Table 5. Post hoc tests between groups for each of the items of the *benefits* variable that reached statistical significance (Bonferroni's test)

Benefits*	G1-G2	G1-G3	G1-G4	G1-G5	G2-G3	G2-G4	G3-G5	G4-G5
Item 1	1.79**	2.74***	2.30***	1.36*			1.38*	
Item 2	1.13*	1.48***	1.24***	1.06*				
Item 3		1.17**					1.22**	0.93*
Item 4		1.56***	1.30***					
Item 5	1.52*	1.97***	1.77***	1.47*				
Item 6		1.26***	1.29***					
Item 7								
Item 8		1.94*						
Item 9		2.33***	2.19***					
Item 10		1.85***	2.07***					
Item 11		1.88***	1.93***					
Item 12		1.80***	1.28*					
Item 13		1.99***	1.98***		1.32**	1.30**	1.43***	1.42***
Item14	1.92***	2.80***	2.74***	1.49**			1.31**	1.25**

G1= Precontemplation; G2= Contemplation; G3= Action; G4= Action-Maintenance; G5= Relapse. * In Appendix 1 the formulation of the items is shown.

Table 6. ANCOVAs for each of the items of the *barriers* variable. Test F and significance level. Means and standard deviations of the items in each of the groups

Barriers*	F	p	G1 N = 24		G2 N = 20		G3 N = 29		G4 N = 56		G5 N = 22	
			X	SD	X	SD	X	SD	X	SD	X	SD
Item 1	2.05	0.06	3.42	2.28	2.00	1.59	1.76	1.85	2.21	2.21	2.64	2.48
Item 2	1.84	0.10	4.25	2.40	2.15	1.39	3.48	2.13	3.73	2.56	3.86	2.62
Item 3	1.03	0.41	3.38	1.64	2.40	1.43	2.62	1.88	2.61	2.21	3.36	2.34
Item 4	3.91	0.00	4.79	2.55	3.65	2.23	3.76	2.36	2.82	2.18	3.59	2.72
Item 5	3.33	0.00	3.92	2.55	2.45	1.79	2.86	2.18	2.46	2.12	3.73	2.68
Item 6	4.22	0.00	4.96	2.37	2.90	2.22	2.59	2.31	2.88	2.54	3.23	2.67
Item 7	7.96	0.00	5.96	1.85	5.65	2.08	3.48	2.28	3.00	2.30	4.68	2.64
Item 8	3.70	0.00	5.21	2.19	4.10	2.25	3.66	2.42	2.95	2.19	4.64	2.34
Item 9	1.12	0.35	4.38	2.00	3.80	1.80	3.69	2.52	3.93	2.53	4.82	2.34
Item 10	3.58	0.00	5.00	2.30	4.40	2.04	4.28	2.36	3.43	2.37	5.32	2.10
Item 11	2.26	0.04	5.29	2.39	4.70	2.34	4.90	2.51	3.77	2.55	5.18	2.34
Item 12	2.55	0.02	2.75	1.75	2.65	1.93	2.79	2.32	2.36	1.95	4.36	2.54
Item 13	3.66	0.00	3.92	1.91	3.00	1.89	3.10	2.60	2.23	2.12	3.50	2.77
Item 14	3.57	0.00	5.50	1.98	3.40	2.30	3.00	2.61	3.32	2.74	4.23	2.43
Item 15	1.92	0.08	2.63	1.56	2.20	1.40	1.83	1.47	2.50	2.22	3.27	2.57
Item 16	1.57	0.16	2.75	1.92	2.40	1.43	2.41	2.03	2.43	2.31	3.86	2.21
Item 17	1.80	0.10	2.50	1.75	2.75	1.83	2.17	2.14	2.43	2.30	4.00	2.55

X = mean. SD= standard deviation. p= significance. The significant information is shaded.
G1= Precontemplation; G2= Contemplation; G3= Action; G4= Action-Maintenance; G5= Relapse
* In Appendix 1 the formulation of the items is shown.

Table 7. Post hoc tests between groups for each of the items of the *barriers* variable that reached statistical significance (Bonferroni's test)

Barriers*	G1-G3	G1-G4	G2-G3	G2-G4	G3-G5	G4-G5
Item 1						
Item 2						
Item 3						
Item 4						
Item 5						
Item 6	2.25**					
Item 7	2.43***	2.68***	2.35**	2.61***		
Item 8		2.07*				
Item 9						
Item 10						1.75*
Item 11						
Item 12						1.96**
Item 13						
Item 14	2.48**	2.00*				
Item 15						
Item 16						
Item 17					1.83*	1.59*

Significance levels: *≤ 0.05; **≤ 0.01; ***≤ 0.001.
G1= Precontemplation; G2= Contemplation; G3= Action; G4= Action-Maintenance; G5= Relapse.
* In Appendix 1 the formulation of the items is shown.

The contemplation group (G2) considers, to a significantly lesser extent compared to action (G3) and action-maintenance/groups (G4), that the mammogram would make it possible to detect cancer in its early stages and thereby increase the possibilities for a cure (item 13). Finally, the relapse group (G5) vs. the action (G3) and action/ maintenance (G4) groups, is significantly less inclined to believe that: the mammogram would make it possible to detect abnormalities and existing lumps (item 3); it would make it possible to detect cancer in its early stage and thus increase possibilities of a cure (item 13); it would also provide health control (item 14). They are less likely to believe that the mammogram would confirm that everything is going well (item 1) in comparison with the action group (G3).

3.3. Differences between Stages in the Perceived Barriers Items

The results of covariance analyses for each item of the perceived barriers variable are shown in Table 6. In Table 7 the contrasts that reached statistical significance (p<.05) are shown. Even though a total of ten out of the seventeen items of the scale show statistically significant differences, only 7 reach statistical significance in post hoc tests, perhaps due to the small size of some of the subgroups (see Table 7).

The results show that differences are mainly established between action (G3) and action/ maintenance (G4) groups in contrast with the rest. Therefore, both groups perceive to a significantly lesser extent than the precontemplation (G1) and contemplation (G2) groups that a mammogram would imply undergoing a test that it is not familiar to them (item 7) and, compared to the relapse group (G5), were not as likely to believe that it would be difficult to have a mammogram if the screening center was more than a few minutes away from home by car (item 17).

Furthermore, women from the action/ maintenance group (G4) vs. the precontemplation group (G1) believe it is less likely that the mammography would imply thinking about the possibility of having breast cancer (item 8) and they would rather not know if they have or do not have breast cancer (item 14). In contrast with the relapse group (G5) they are less inclined to think that the mammography would make them feel anxious (item 10) or that it would be difficult for them to have a mammography because they are always very busy (item 12).

The action group (G3) is less likely to believe that the mammogram is not convenient in their case (item 6) or they would rather not know if they have or do not have breast cancer (item 14), which is significantly different from the precontemplation group (G1).

3.4. Differences between Stages and Items of the Information Scale

In the covariance analyses (Table 8), all items in the information scale showed statistically significant differences according to the mammography stage, although some of them did not reach statistical significance in contrast to post hoc tests between groups (Table 9).

The results show that the precontemplation (G1) and relapse (G5) groups are the ones which have less information about the techniques of early breast cancer detection. Both groups, in contrast with the action (G3) and action/maintenance (G4) groups are not as informed about the need to have mammograms in the absence of symptoms (item 4); the need to continue screening from a certain age even though nothing abnormal is found (item 6); and the need to have mammograms at their age (item 9). In addition, the precontemplation group (G1) vs. the action (G3) and action/maintenance (G4) groups are less likely to be aware that the mammogram is a useful method for women of their age (item 1) and that from a certain age it is necessary for women to have periodic mammograms (item 3).

It is worth noting that the contemplation group (G2), compared to the action (G3) and action/maintenance (G4) groups, is significantly less aware that at their age it is necessary to have mammograms (item 9) and, although only in contrast with the action group (G3), that from a certain age it is necessary that women have periodical mammograms (item 3).

CONCLUSIONS

In this study we have considered five groups of women defined according to the stage of mammography adoption (precontemplation, contemplation, action, action/maintenance, and relapse), contrasting them in a series of variables postulated as predictors of health behaviors on behalf of sociocognitive models: general health motivation, perceived susceptibility to breast cancer, perceived severity of this illness, perceived benefits and barriers of the mammogram, perceived social pressure to undergo this technique, perceived control over it, and the degree of information about breast cancer screening. The results have proved how all these variables, except "susceptibility" and "severity", establish statistically significant differences between some of the considered stages—the "benefits" variable is the one that distinguishes between a greater number of stages.

Regarding perceived susceptibility, it is worth noting that even though no statistically significant differences have been found depending on the stage of mammography adoption, the results show that the women in the precontemplation stage (they have never had a mammography or have no intention to have it done) have a greater perceived susceptibility to breast cancer. A result which goes against what was theoretically postulated by the

Health Belief Model and which has a bearing on the weakness of the empirical results shown in the bibliography regarding the perceived susceptibility to breast cancer as a predictor of the adoption of preventative behaviors in this illness (Andreu, Galdón and Durá, 2001; Champion, 1994; Lerman, Rimer, Trock, Balshem and Engstrom, 1990; Skinner et al., 1998a; Vaile et al., 1993). Even though the variable of perceived severity of breast cancer reaches statistical significance in the multivaried analysis, in the contrasts between stage groups it does not. This result may be due to the small size of the sample of some subgroups, but it is also true that it is a variable with scarce presence in studies analyzing the mammography behavior and the results are not very consistent either (Andreu et al., 2001; Champion, 1994; Glanz, Rimer, Lerman and McGovern, 1992; Montano and Taplin, 1991; Stein et al., 1992; Vernon, Laville and Jackson, 1990); in fact, in research carried out in Spain, it is the only variable associated with attendance at a mammographic screening program in a contrary way to the proposal by the Health Belief Model, which means inhibiting participation (Galdón, Durá, Andreu and Tuells, 2000).

The results in the case of the rest of the variables not only reach statistical significance but they also do it in the theoretically expected direction, all of which are positively associated with the stages that are mostly involved with mammography behavior. Thus, women who do not even have the intention to have a mammography (precontemplation stage) show significantly less general health motivation, less information about early detection techniques of breast cancer; they perceive more barriers and fewer benefits from the screening and perceive less control over this preventative behavior than women who meet or intend to meet the recommended screening guidelines again (action and action/maintenance stages). In the social pressure variable, even though it only distinguishes between the precontemplation and action stage, the results are also along the lines of what is theoretically expected; the first ones perceiving less social pressure to undergo screening. Finally, it is worth pointing out that some of these variables also distinguish between women who meet or intend to meet the recommended repeated screening guidelines and those who have abandoned mammograms (relapse group), the latter showing less information about the early detection techniques for breast cancer and perceiving more barriers and fewer benefits of screening.

Table 8. ANCOVAs for each of the items of the *information* variable. Test F and significance level. Means and standard deviations of the items in each of the group

Informacíon*	F	p	G1 N = 24		G2 N = 20		G3 N = 29		G4 N = 56		G5 N = 22	
			X	SD	X	SD	X	SD	X	SD	X	SD
Item 1	7.22	0.00	0.63	0.50	0.90	0.31	0.97	0.19	1.00	0.00	0.86	0.35
Item 2	2.47	0.03	0.63	0.50	0.70	0.47	0.79	0.41	0.86	0.35	0.73	0.46
Item 3	9.98	0.00	0.54	0.51	0.80	0.41	1.00	0.00	1.00	0.00	0.82	0.40
Item 4	8.24	0.00	0.42	0.50	0.75	0.44	0.90	0.31	0.93	0.26	0.55	0.51
Item 5	7.07	0.00	0.53	0.43	0.68	0.35	0.64	0.33	0.76	0.33	0.51	0.31
Item 6	7.31	0.00	0.58	0.50	0.85	0.37	0.97	0.19	1.00	0.00	0.73	0.46
Item 7	3.98	0.00	0.50	0.51	0.65	0.49	0.45	0.51	0.59	0.50	0.27	0.46
Item 8	5.18	0.00	0.46	0.51	0.75	0.44	0.52	0.51	0.57	0.50	0.32	0.48
Item 9	11.34	0.00	0.42	0.50	0.75	0.44	0.97	0.19	0.98	0.13	0.68	0.39

X = mean. SD= standard deviation. p= significance. The significant information is shaded.
G1= Precontemplation; G2= Contemplation; G3= Action; G4= Action-Maintenance; G5= Relapse.
* In Appendix 1 the formulation of the items is shown.

Table 9. Post hoc tests between groups for each of the items of the *information* variable that reached statistical significance (Bonferroni's test)

Information*	G1-G3	G1-G4	G1-G5	G2-G3	G2-G4	G3-G5	G4-G5
Item 1	0.33***	0.32***					
Item 2							
Item 3	0.44***	0.40***	0.24*	0.26*			
Item 4	0.47***	0.44***				0.38**	0.35**
Item 5							
Item 6	0.37***	0.37***				0.25*	0.25*
Item 7							
Item 8					0.25*		
Item 9	0.53***	0.50***		0.28*		0.30*	0.27*

Significance levels: *≤ 0.05; **≤ 0.01; ***≤ 0.001

G1= Precontemplation; G2= Contemplation; G3= Action; G4= Action-Maintenance; G5= Relapse

* In Appendix 1 the formulation of the items is shown.

These results are also along the lines of others found in different empirical studies that, as we have already mentioned, have used the constructs from the transtheoretical model or have used the variables of the Health Belief Model to distinguish between mammography stages (Brenes and Skinner, 1999; Chamot et al., 2001; Champion, 1994; Champion and Skinner, 2003; Champion and Springston, 1999; Clark, et al., 1998; Rakowski et al., 1992, 1993; 1996; 1997a, 1997b; Rimer et al., 1996; Skinner et al., 1997, 1998a; Stoddard et al., 1998). Also other research in which a specific model is not adopted but the relation of certain sociocognitive variables with the stages of the mammography adoption are analyzed, indicate similar results; such is the case of the variable of general health motivation (Campbell et al., 2000) or the received social pressure to undergo screening (Mah and Bryant, 1997; Pearlman et al., 1997; Pearlman, Rakowski and Ehrich, 1995; Stoddard et al., 1998).

The analysis of the specific items in the information scale has made it possible to know more specifically the type of information associated with meeting recommended screening guidelines. Thus, women who do not have mammograms or do not have the intention to have them (precontemplation) differ from those who do have them (action and action/maintenance groups): they are unaware of (i) the age interval in which it is necessary to be screened; (ii) the need to have them from a certain age and periodically; and (iii) that even though there are no symptoms or the mammogram does not detect anything abnormal, screenings are still necessary. Women who stop attending screening (relapse) differ from those who have the intention to continue attending or continue attending (action and action/maintenance) in the ignorance of the suitable age to have mammograms and must continue to be screened even though there are no abnormalities in the breast or the mammogram does not show anything abnormal.

Even though the information variable is not the principal predictor of mammography behavior, neither from the belief models (Health Belief Model and Theory of Planned Behavior) nor from the stages model (Transtheoretical Model), the empirical evidence shows that the information about breast cancer and mammography screening is positively associated with the use of this technique (Fajardo, Saint-Germain, Meakem, Rose and Hillman, 1992; O'Connor and Perrault, 1995). More specifically, research shows that knowledge of what a mammogram is and its purpose is necessary for women to meet the recommended guidelines although it does not guarantee its practice (Glanz et al., 1992). Likewise, other research shows that it is particularly important to know the need for periodical screening even when there are no symptoms (Donato et al. 1991; Durá, Andreu, Galdón and Tuells, 2004; Kee, Telford, Donaghy and O'Doherty, 1992; Munn, 1993). Our study, as we have pointed out, confirms these results.

Finally, we will focus more specifically on the results found for the items of perceived benefits and barriers scales of the mammography screening since, from the perspective of stages of change models and more specifically from the Transtheoretical Model, great importance is given to these types of beliefs. We know that it is the cognitive analysis of costs-benefits, which is associated with behavioral change. In other words, the decisional balance is the one which distinguishes between the different stages of mammography adoption as empirical studies prove (Champion, 1994; Champion et al., 2003; Champion and Springston, 1999; Clark et al., 1998; Clark et al. 2002; Lauver et al., 2003; Rakowski et a., 1993; Rakowski et al., 1996; Rakowski et al., 1997a, 1997b; Rakowski et al., 1998; Rimer et al., 1996; Skinner et al., 1997; Skinner et al. 1998b; Spencer et al., 2005; Stoddard et al., 1998).

There are two benefit items that best distinguish between the different stages of mammography adoption: one referred to the clinical effectiveness of the mammogram and another referred to the emotional benefit associated with the perception of better health control making this technique possible. The belief that screening increases the possibilities of breast cancer treatment by detecting the illness early differentiates women who continue attending screening (action and action/maintenance) from those who have never had a mammography (precontemplation and contemplation) or have stopped (relapse). Not believing that periodical screening provides health control is what specifically characterizes women who have never had a mammogram and do not even have the intention to have one in the future, contrary to the rest. The perception of both clinical and emotional benefits is a variable systematically associated with attending screening and with the adoption of stages more implicated in this preventative behavior (Bauman, Brown, Fontana and Cameron, 1993; Champion and Miller, 1996; Champion, 1994; Champion et al., 2003; Champion and Skinner, 2003; Lostao, Chorot, Sandín and Lacabe 1996; Skinner et al., 1997; Vernon et al., 1990). Our results point out that these benefits have the capacity to distinguish even between the two least engaged stages of mammography behavior (precontemplation and contemplation), associating a better perception of clinical and emotional benefits with the intention to undergo mammography screening in the future.

Another significant result in relation to the perceived benefits of the mammogram is item 6 of the scale (the mammogram "would enable the detection of a cancer that I could not have found with breast self-examination") which distinguishes the precontemplation group from the action and action/maintenance groups. Thus, women who have never had a mammogram or do not intend to have one believe that breast self-examination has the same clinical effectiveness as the mammogram; perhaps this false belief may be dissuading them from having it done.

Regarding the beliefs mentioned in perceived barriers to mammography screening, it is worth noting that the item that specifically distinguishes between the least engaged stages to mammography adoption (precontemplation and contemplation) in contrast with the most engaged (action and action/maintenance) is the one mentioned in the perception of familiarity with the mammogram. Therefore, and along the lines of the results found in the study by Champion and Springston (1999), the lack of familiarity with the test differentiates women who have never undergone a screening. This result is notable since it shows the need to make it known to all women who should undergo mammograms and they still have not, certain aspects related to the mammography procedure itself (the place where it is performed, what the mammography technique consists of, the necessary time, etc.) with the aim that they become familiar with the procedure and not letting their ignorance dissuade them from undergoing screening.

Moreover, women in the least engaged stage of mammography behavior (precontemplation) perceive to a significantly higher degree than those that meet the guidelines (action/maintenance) or have the intention to keep meeting the guidelines (action), several emotionally-related barriers, mainly, worry and fear that they associate with mammograms and breast cancer; for example, they would rather not know if they have or do not have breast cancer. Precisely these emotional barriers play a very important role, according to our results, in the case of women who do not meet the recommended screening guidelines anymore or have decided not to undergo a repeated mammography screening (relapse): women who suffer a relapse represent more fear and anxiety facing a mammography as a test in itself. Champion and Skinner (2003) show some similar results in which emotional barriers distinguished between the women from contemplation groups and the ones from action and relapse groups. Similarly, Skinner et al. (1998b) reported that women in contemplation showed higher scores in the barriers associated with fear of mammograms.

To conclude, it is worth noting that women who are in the relapse stage are the ones who differ from women who keep attending screenings (action and/or action/maintenance) in beliefs related to practical obstacles (such as lack of time to attend mammography screenings or the distance of the screening center). These results also coincide with the ones found in other studies in which these types of barriers distinguished between the women from the most engaged stage and the rest (Skinner et al. 1997). Regarding these practical obstacles it should be pointed out that, even though some studies show that the perception of a mammography as something painful is one of the barriers that women in the precontemplation and contemplation stages put forward most strongly (Skinner et al. 1997, 1998b), our results coincide contrarily with the ones found in another Spanish sample (Durá et al. 2004) showing that the belief that a mammography can be painful is not a significant predictor of mammography behavior.

To finish this chapter we want to emphasize that the knowledge of all these results prove notable when it comes to associating beliefs to the processes-of-change and to the adoption of cancer screening behavior: the change in individuals' beliefs makes changes in terms of behavior. Therefore, the results of our study have great applicability when it comes to designing public health campaign devoted to breast cancer prevention. It proves very important to be able to get an idea of what types of beliefs towards mammography and breast cancer have a higher or lower specific importance, since it means that we are able to elaborate messages and interventions adapted to the need of every subgroup. For instance, they can be used to individually design appointment reminders that are sent to women by mail according to the stage they are in, taking into account the reasons given by women who have never had a mammogram and do not think about having it done it, or the motives of those who have had them but stop attending the breast cancer prevention program.

Therefore, our results clearly show that, for women who have never had mammograms or do not even think about having it done (precontemplation stage), it is essential to inform them of the importance of health value and to inform them about the mammography as a technique of early breast cancer detection (mainly the need of its regular practice from a certain age and in absence of symptoms). They should also be made aware of the advantages of this technique, not only in terms of the clinical effectiveness in the diagnosis and cancer treatment, but also at the emotional level (for the peace of mind brought about by a negative result in the test), and counteract the possible perceived disadvantages of this technique informing them about the mammography procedure (what it consists of, how is performed, how long it takes, etc.), with the aim of increasing the familiarity with the technique and perceived control over it. Our results also show that it is necessary to involve social agents who can exert pressure so that women will undergo screening, for example, through the health system (general physician) or through the media (television, press, radio, etc.). It is worth noting that, of all these variables, it seems that the perception of associated benefits of the mammography is the most outstanding, since our results show that this variable will lead women who have never had a mammography to actually having the intention to have one in the future (contemplation).

When women have already undergone mammography screening, and with the aim of not abandoning such a practice, it is necessary, according to our results, to keep transmitting information about the advantage of undergoing screening from a certain age even in the absence of symptoms, highlighting the benefits of the mammography to control breast cancer, and counteract the possible perceived disadvantages of mammography screening, mainly the ones related to practical obstacles (distance from the screening centre, waste of time, etc.)

All this will have a direct consequence on participation levels, which is after all the last and necessary objective of all the campaigns stressing early detection of breast cancer. Knowing the beliefs that are significantly related to the stages-of-adoption and taking them into account, we can promote a behavioral change in which women move along the stages in the continuum from the least engaged stages of mammography adoption (precontemplation and contemplation) to the most engaged (action and action/maintenance), and avoid abandoning mammography screening (relapse stage). Some studies have already applied interventions on the matter with promising results (Champion et al., 2003; Clark et al., 2002; Rakowski et al., 1998).

We do not want to close this chapter without acknowledging some limitations of the study mainly related to our sample size. Given that the total sample had to be subdivided into five subgroups according to the stage of the mammography adoption, the size of some subgroups is relatively small; which could have been the reason why some comparisons did not reach a level of statistical significance. However it is necessary to emphasize that the different size of the groups is representative of the population. Therefore, and as we have already mentioned, the sample was obtained mainly from associations in which the organization itself encouraged attending mammography screenings, thereby achieving the goal that most of them are in the action and action/maintenance stages of mammography behavior. In any case, the results obtained from this study encourage empirically researching the validity of the application of the Transtheoretical Model to cancer screening behavior; a matter of great social and scientific importance (Spencer, Pagell and Adams, 2005).

APPENDIX 1

Benefits Items MAMMOGRAPHY:	Barriers Items MAMMOGRAPHY:	Information Items
Item 1: It would confirm that everything is going well	Item 1: It would be a waste of time	Item 1: A mammography is a useful method for women of my age.
Item 2: It would enable an early breast cancer diagnosis if I had it	Item 2: It would be uncomfortable or unpleasant	Item 2: A woman may have breast cancer even if she presents no symptoms or does not feel ill.
Item 3: It would enable the detection of abnormalities and non-cancerous lumps if I had them	Item 3: It would possibly be detrimental due to X-rays	Item 3: From a certain age it is necessary for women to have periodical mammographies done.
Item 4: It would enable an early treatment if I had something wrong	Item 4: It would make me worry needlessly	Item 4: A woman only needs to have a mammography when she finds something abnormal.
Item 5: It would confirm that nothing is wrong	Item 5: It would be embarrassing or shameful for me	Item 5: Some abnormal changes in the breast include: secretion, a lump, a dimple or all.
Item 6: It would enable the detection of a cancer that I could not have found with breast self examination	Item 6 : It would not seem convenient to me in my case	Item 6: From a certain age it is necessary for women to have mammographies even if nothing abnormal is detected.
Item 7: It would enable the detection of a cancer that could not be detected by means of physical examination	Item 7: It would imply taking a test that I am not familiar with	Item 7: If I have had a smear test this year I do not need to have a mammography.
Item 8: My possibility of dieing of breast cancer would decrease	Item 8: It would imply thinking about the possibility that I may have cancer	Item 8: If a woman has already had a couple of mammographies, she does not need anymore.
Item 9: It would help me stop worrying about my health every year or so	Item 9: It could be painful	Item 9: At my age it is necessary to have mammographies.
Item 10: It would help me take my mind of it	Item 10: It would make me feel anxious	

APPENDIX 1 (CONTINUED)

Benefits Items MAMMOGRAPHY:	Barriers Items MAMMOGRAPHY:	Information Items
Item 11: As a routine, I would stop worrying about the state of my health	Item 11: I would be afraid if something abnormal were found	
Item 12: It would make the treatment not look so bad for having detected the breast cancer early	Item 12: It would be difficult because I am always very busy	
Item 13: It would enable the detection of breast cancer at an early stage, thus increasing the number of possibilities for cure	Item 13: It is useless because if something abnormal is found there will be no remedy	
Item 14: It would often provide me with control over my health	Item 14: I prefer not to know if I have breast cancer or not	
	Item 15: It would take up too much of my time	
	Item 16: It would be difficult, because I do not remember how to make an appointment	
	Item 17: It would be hard, if the place to have it were more than a few minutes away from home	

REFERENCES

Agency for Healthcare Research and Quality. (2002). *Screening for Breast Cancer. Recommendation and Rationale.* URL available: http://www. ahrq.gov/clinic/
3rduspstf/breastcancer/brcanrr.htm.

Ajzen, Y. (1988). *Attitudes, personality, and behavior.* Chicago: The Dorsey Press.

Ajzen, Y. (1991). The Theory of Planned Behavior. *Organizational Behavior and Human Decision Processes,* 50: 179-211.

Ajzen, Y., and Fishbein, M. (1980): *Understanding attitudes and predicting social behavior.* Englewood Cliffs, N.J.: Prentice Hall.

Andreu, Y., Galdon, Mª J., and Durá, E. (2001). Prevención secundaria del cáncer de mama: el papel de las creencias de salud. In M.R. Dias and E. Durá (coords.), *Territorios da Psicología Oncológica* (547-578). Lisboa: Climepsi Editores.

Bandura, A. (1977). Self-efficacy: toward a unifying theory of behaviour change. *Psychological Review, 84,* 191-215.

Bandura, A. (1997). *Self-efficacy: The exercise of control.* New York: Freeman.

Bauman, L., Brown, R., Fontana, A., and Cameron, L. (1993). Testing a model of mammography intention. *Journal of Applied Social Psychology, 23,*1733-1756.

Becker, M.H. (1974). The health belief model and sick role behavior. *Health Education Monographs, 2,* 409-419.

Brenes, G.A., and Skinner, C.S. (1999). Psychological factors related to stage of mammography adoption. *J* Womens Health Gend Based Med. *8,* 1313-21.

Campbell, M.K., Tessaro, I., DeVellis, B., Benedict, S., Kelsey, K., Belton, L., and Henriquez-Roldan, C. (2000). Tailoring and targeting a worksite health promotion program to address multiple health behaviour among blue-collar women. *American Journal of Health Promotion, 14,* 306-313.

Chamot, E., Charvet, A.I., and Perneger, T.V. (2001). Predicting stages of adoption of mammography screening in a general population. *European Journal of Cancer, 37,* 1869-77.

Champion, V. (1993). Instrument refinement for breast cancer screening behaviours. *Nursing Reserch, 42,* 139-143.

Champion, V. (1994). Beliefs about breast cancer and mammography by behavioural stage. *Oncology Nursing Forum, 21,* 1009-1014.

Champion, V., Maraj, M., Hui, S., Perkins, A.J., Tierney, W., Menon, U., and Skinner, C.S. (2003). Comparisons of tailored interventions to increase mammography screening in nonadherent older women. *Preventive Medicine, 36,* 150-158.

Champion, V., and Miller, T. (1996). Predicting mammography utilization through model generation. *Psychology, Health and Medicine, 1,* 273-283.

Champion, V., and Skinner, C.S. (2003). Differences in perceptions of risk, benefits and barriers by stage of mammography adoption. *Journal of Women's Health, 12,* 277-286.

Champion, V., and Springston, J. (1999). Mammography adherence and beliefs in a sample of low-income African American women. *International Journal of Behavioral Medicine, 6,* 228-240.

Clark, M.A., Rakowski, W., Ehrich, B., Pearlman, D.N., Goldstein, M.G., Dube, C.E., Rimer, B.K., and Woolverton, H. (1998). Stages of adopting regular screening mammography. Do women differ in decisional balance within stages?. *Journal of Health Psychology, 3,* 491-506.

Clark, M.A., Rakowski, W., Ehrich, B., Rimer, B.K., Velicer, W.F., Dube, C.E., Pearlman, D.N., Peterson, K.K., and Goldstein, M.G. (2002). The effect of a stage-matched and tailores intervention on repeat mammography. *American Journal of Preventive Medicine, 22,* 1-7.

Conner, M., and Norman, P. (2001). Health Behavior. In D. Johnston and M. Johnston (eds.), *Health Psychology, Vol. 8. Comprehensive Clinical Psychology* (pp. 1-37*).* Amsterdam: Elsevier.

Crane L.A., Leakey, T.A., Ehrsam, G., et al. (2000). Effectiveness and cost-effectiveness of multiple outcalls to promote mammography among low-income women. *Cancer Epidemiology Biomarkers and Prevention, 9,* 923-931.

Deck, W., and Kakuma, R. (2005). *Mammographie de dépistage: une réévaluation.* Québec: AETMIS.

Di Clemente, C.C., and Hughes, S.L. (1990). Stages of change profiles in alcoholism treatment. *Journal of Substance Abuse, 2,* 217-235.

Donato, F., Bollani, A., Spiazzi, R., Soldo, M., Pasquale, L., Monarca, S., Lucini, L., and Nardi, G. (1991). Factors associated with non-participation of women in a breast cancer screening program in a town in northern Italy. *Journal of Epidemiology and Community Health, 45,* 59-64.

Durá, E., Andreu, Y., and Galdón, MªJ. (2001). Aplicación de los modelos sociocognitivos a la prevención secundaria del cáncer de mama. *Psicología Conductual, 9,* 99-130.

Durá, E., Andreu, Y., Galdón, M.J., and Tuells, J. (2004). Razones de no asistencia a un programa de cribado mamográfico. *Psicooncología, 1,* 31-50.

Fajardo, L.L., Saint-Germain, M., Meakem, T.J., Rose, C., and Hillman, B.J. (1992). Factors influencing women to undergo screening mammography. *Radiology, 184,* 59-63.

Galdón, MªJ., Durá, E., Andreu, Y., and Tuells, J. (2000). Creencias de salud relacionadas con la participación en un programa de cribado mamográfico. *Psicología Conductual, 8,* 357-373.

Galdón, MªJ., Durá, E., Andreu, Y. , Tuells, E., and Ibáñez, E. (2003). La detección temprana del cáncer de mama: creencias de salud y cribado mamográfico. *Revista de Psicología. Universitas Tarraconenis, XXV,* 8-22.

Glanz, K., Rimer, B.K., Lerman, C., and McGovern, P. (1992). Factors influencing acceptance of mammography: Implications for enhancing worksite cancer control. *American Journal of Health Promotion, 7,* 28-37.

Gotzsche, P.C., and Olsen, O. (2000). Is screening for breast cancer with mammography justifiable?. *Lancet, 355,* 129-34.

Hair, J.F., Anderson, R.E., Tatham, R.L., and Black, W.C. (1999). *Análisis Multivariante.* Madrid: Prentice Hall Iberia.

Humphrey, L.L., Helfand, M., Chan, B.K., and Woolf, S.H. (2002). Breast cancer screening: a summary of the evidence for the U.S. Preventive Services Task Force. *Annals of Internal Medicine, 137,* 347-360.

Kee, F., Telford, A.M., Donaghy, P., and O'Doherty, A. (1992). Attitude or access: reasons for not attending mammography in Northern Ireland. *European Journal of Cancer Prevention, 1,* 311-315.

Kerlikowske, K., Grady, D., Rubin, S.M., Sandrock, C., and Ernster, V.L. (1995). Efficacy of screening mammography. A meta-analysis. *JAMA, 273,*149-154.

Lauver, D.R., Henriques, J.B., Settersten, L., and Bumann, M.C. (2003). Psychosocial variables, external barriers and stage of mammography adoption. *Health Psychology, 22,* 649-653.

Lerman, C., Rimer, B., Trock, B., Balshem, A., and Engstrom, P.F. (1990). Factors associated with repeat adherence to breast cancer screening. *Preventive Medicine, 19,* 279-290.

Lipkus, I.M., Rimer, B.K., Halabi, S., and Strigo, T.S. (2000). Can tailored interventions increase mammography use among HMO women?. *American Journal of Preventive Medicine, 18,* 1-10.

Lostao, L., Chorot, P., Sandín, B., and Lacabe, F. (1996). Variables psicosociales relacionadas con la participación en un "screening" de cáncer de mama. *Arbor CLIV, 608,* 33-71.

McCance, K. L., Mooney, K. H., Smith, K. R., and Field, R. (1990). Validity and reliability of a breast cancer knowledge test. *American Journal of Preventive Medicine, 6,* 93-98.

Mah, Z., and Bryant, H.E. (1997). The role of past mammography and future intentions in screening mammography use. *Cancer Detection and Prevention, 21,* 213-220.

Marteau, T.M. (1994). Psychology and screening: Narrowing the gap between efficacy and effectiveness. *British Journal of Clinical Psychology, 33,* 1-10.

Meystre-Agustoni, G., Dubois-Arber, F., Landstheer, J.P., and Paccaud, F. (1998). Exploring the reasons for non-participation of women in a breast cancer screening campaign. *European Journal of Public Health, 8,* 143-145.

Miller, A.B., To, T., Baines, C.J., and Wall, C. (2002). The Canadian National Breast Screening Study-1: breast cancer mortality after 11 to 16 years of follow-up. A randomized screening trial of mammography in women aged 40 to 49 years. *Annals of Internal Medicine, 137,* 305-312.

Montano, D.E., and Taplin, S.H. (1991). A test of an expanded theory of reasoned action to predict mammography participation. *Social Science Medicine, 32,* 733-741.

Munn, E.M. (1993). Nonparticipation in mammography screening: apathy, anxiety or cost?. *New Zealand Medical Journal, 106,* 284-286.

Nystrom, L., Andersson, I., Bjurstam, N., Frisell, J., Nordenskjold, B., and Rutqvist, L.E. (2002). Long-term effects of mammography screening: updated overview of the Swedish randomised trials. *Lancet, 359,* 909-919.

O'Connor, A., and Perrault, D. (1995). Importance of physician's role highlighted in survey of women's breast screening practices. *Canadian Journal of Public Health, 86,* 42-45.

Olsen, O., and Gotzsche, P.C. (2001): Cochrane review on screening for breast cancer with mammography. *Lancet, 358,* 1340-1342.

Pearlman, D.N., Rakowski, W., Clark, M.A., et al. (1997). Why do women's attitudes toward mammography change over time?. Implications for physician-patient communication. *Cancer Epidemiology Biomarker Prevention, 6,* 451-457.

Pearlman, D.N., Rakowski, W, and Ehrich, B. (1995). The information environment of women and mammography screening: assessing reciprocity in social relationships. *Clinical Journal of Women's Health, 4,* 541-553.

Pelfrene, E.R., Bleyen, L.J., and Backer, G. (1998). Uptake in breast cancer screening: A sociogeographical analysis. *European Journal of Public Health, 8,* 146-149.

Primic-Zakelj, M. (1999). Screening mammography for early detection of breast cancer. *Annals of Oncology, 19,* 121-127.

Prochaska, J.O., and Diclemente, C.C. (1982). Tanstheoretical therapy: Toward a more integrative model of change. *Psychotherapy: Theory, Research and Practice, 20,* 161-173.

Prochaska, J.O., and Diclemente, C.C. (1983). Stages and processes of self-change in smoking: Toward and integrative model of change. *Journal of Consulting and Clinical Psychology, 5,* 390-395.

Rakowski, W., Dube, C.E., Marcus, B.H., Prochaska, J.O., Velicer, W.F., and Abrams, D.B. (1992). Assessing elements of women's decisions about mammography. *Health Psychology, 11,* 111-118.

Rakowski, W., Fulton, J.P., and Feldman, J.P. (1993). Women's decision making about mammography: A replication of the relationship between stages of adoption and decisional balance. *Health Psychology, 12,* 209-214.

Rakowski, W., Ehrich, B., Dube, C.E., Pearlman, D.N., Goldstein, M.G., Peterson, K.K., Rimer, B.K., and Woolverton, H. (1996). Screening mammography and constructs from the Transtheoretical model: associations using two definitions of the stages of adoption. *Annals of Behavioral Medecine, 18,* 91-100.

Rakowski, W., Andersen, M.R., Stoddard, A.M., Urban, N., Rimer, B.K., Lane, D.S., Fox, S.A., and Costanza, M.E. (1997a). Confirmatory analysis of opinions regarding the pros and cons of mammography. *Health Psychology, 16,* 433-441.

Rakowski, W., Clark, M.A.; Pearlman, D.N.; Ehrich, B.; Rimer, B.K.; Goldstein, M.G.; Dube, C.E., and Woolverton, H. (1997b). Integrating pros and cons for mammography and Pap testing: extending the construct of decisional balance to two behaviors. *Preventive Medecine, 26,* 664-673.

Rakowski, W., Ehrich, B., Goldstein, M.G., Rimer, B.K., Pearlman, D.N., Clark, M.A., Velicer, W.F., and Woolverton, H. (1998). Increasing mammography among women aged 40-74 by use of a stage-matched, tailored intervention. *Preventive Medecine, 27,* 748-756.

Rimer B.K., Conaway, M.R., Lyna P.R., et al. (1996). Cancer screening practices among women in a community health center population. *American Journal of Preventive Medicine, 12,* 351-357.

Rimer, B.K., Halabi, S., Skinner, C.S., et al. (2001). The short-term impact of tailored mammography decision-making interventions. *Patient Educ Counseling, 1429,* 1-17.

Ringash, J., and The Canadian Task Force on Preventive Health Care. (2001). Preventive health care, 2001 update: screening mammography among women aged 40-49 years at average risk of breast cancer. *Canadian Medical Association Journal, 164,* 469-76.

Rippon, M.B. (1994). Breast Cancer: Early detection and prevention. *Cancer Researcher Weekly, 2,* 17.

Rosenstock, I.M. (1966). Why people use health services?. *Milbank Memorial Fund Quartely, 44,* 94-121.

Rosenstock, I.M. (1990). The health belief model: Explaining health behavior through expectancies. In K. Glanz, F.M. Lewis, and B.K Rimer (eds.), *Health Behavior and Health Education. Theory, Research and Practice* (39-62). San Francisco: Jossey Bass Publishers.

Rosenstock, I.M., Strecher, V., and Becker, M.R. (1988). Social Learning Learning Theory and the Health Belief Model. *Health Education Quarterly, 15,* 175-183.

Sheeran, P., and Abraham, C. (1996). The Health Belief Model. In M. Conner, and P. Norman (eds.), *Predicting Health Behavior* (pp. 23-61). Buckingham, UK: Open University Press.

Skinner, C., Strecher, V., and Hospers, H. (1994). Physicians′ recommendations for mammography: do tailored messages make a difference? *American Journal of Public Heatlh, 84,* 43-49.

Skinner, C.S., Champion, V., Gonin, R., and Hanna, M. (1997). Do perceived barriers and benefits vary by mammography stage?. *Psychology, Health and Medicine, 2,* 65-75.

Skinner, C.S., Kreuter, M.W., Kobrin, S., and Strecher, V.J. (1998a). Perceived and actual breast cancer risk: Optimistic and pessimistic biases. *Journal of Health Psychology, 3,* 181-193.

Skinner, C.S., Arfken, C.L., and Sykes, R.K. (1998b). Knowledge, perceptions and mammography stage of adoption among older urban women. *American Journal of Preventive Medicine, 14,* 54-63.

Sox, H. (2002). Screening mammography for younger women: back to basics. *Annals of Internal Medicine, 137,* 361-362.

Spencer, L., Pagell, F., and Adams, T. (2005). Applying the Transtheoretical Model to cancer screening behavior. *American Journal of Health Behaviour, 29,* 36-56.

Stein, J.A., Fox, S.A., Murata, P.J., and Morisky, D.E. (1992). Mammography usage and the health belief model. *Health Education Quarterly, 19,* 447-462.

Stillman, M.J. (1977). Women's health beliefs about breast cancer and breast self-examination to secondary prevention of breast cancer. *Nursing Research, 6,* 121-127.

Stoddard, A.M.; Rimer, B.K.; Lane, D. et al., (1998). Underusers of mammogram screening: stage of adoption in five U.S. subpopulations. *American Journal of Preventive Medicine, 27,* 478-487.

Vaile, M.S.B., Calnan, M., Rutter, D.R, and Wall, R (1993). Breast cancer screening services in three areas: Uptake and satisfaction. *Journal of Public Health Medicine, 15,* 37-45.

Vernon, S.W., Laville, E.A., and Jackson, G.L. (1990). Participation in breast cancer screening programs: A review. *Social Science Medicine, 30,* 1107-1118.

Wallston, K.A. (1992). Hocus-pocus, the focus isn't strictly on locus: Rotter's social learning theory modified for health. *Cognitive Therapy and Research, 16,* 183-99.

Weinstein, N.D. (1988). The precaution adoption process. *Health Psychology, 7,* 355-386.

In: Breast Cancer Screening and Prevention   ISBN 978-1-61209-288-1
Editor: Jonathan D. Pegg   © 2011 Nova Science Publishers, Inc.

Chapter 3

BREAST CANCER PERCEPTIONS, KNOWLEDGE AND BEHAVIORAL PRACTICES AMONG WOMEN LIVING IN A RURAL COMMUNITY

Saleh M. M. Rahman[*1] *and Selina Rahman*[2]

[1]Behavioral Sciences and Health Education, Institute of Public Health, Florida A and M University, College of Pharmacy and Pharmaceutical Sciences, 209-A FSH Science Research Center, Tallahassee, FL 32307.
[2]Post Doctoral Research Fellow, Environmental Sciences Institute, Adjunct Faculty, Institute of Public Health, Florida A and M University

ABSTRACT

We performed this study to assess women's perceptions, knowledge and behavioral practices for breast cancer prevention in a rural setting. A

[*] Corresponding author: MBBS, PhD, MPH, Assistant Professor, Behavioral Sciences and Health Education, Institute of Public Health, Florida A and M University, College of Pharmacy and Pharmaceutical Sciences, 209-A FSH Science Research Center, Tallahassee, FL 32307. Ph: 850-599-8840. Fax: 850-599-8830. E-mail: saleh.rahman@famu.edu

61-item questionnaire was developed based on Health Belief Model constructs and completed by 185 women age 35 and older. Results showed significant differences in several areas including perceived susceptibility and severity. Overall knowledge was poor. In logistic regression perceived barriers and yearly clinical breast examination appeared to be significant predictors for regular screening behavior (OR=0.02, CI=0.03-0.09 and OR=0.23, CI=0.05-0.99, respectively). Behavioral interventions targeting barriers for rural women need to be designed to include consideration of specific barriers and clear information on the need for regular screening.

Keywords: Breast cancer, perceptions, knowledge and rural women.

INTRODUCTION

An abundance of evidence suggests that there are clear disparities in utilization of preventive services by rural populations. A study based on Behavioral Risk Factor Surveillance showed that women residing in nonmetropolitan areas were less likely to receive mammograms or Pap smears in accordance with recommended guidelines than their urban counterparts (Casey, Call, and Klinger, 2001). Similar findings are also shown in studies based on Medicare Current Beneficiaries Survey (Stearns et al., 2000) and the National Health Interview Survey (Zhang, Tao, and Irwin, 2000). Underutilization of preventive health care services may result in a failure of identifying health problems in time and missing opportunities to reduce mortality or morbidity. A review of cancer incidence in rural versus urban populations found that cancer tends to be diagnosed at more advanced stages among rural populations (Monroe, Ricketts, and Savitz, 1992; Liff, Chow, and Greenburg, 1991), suggesting that rural residents are less likely to receive timely cancer screening tests. In addition, rural residence has been found to be a strong predictor of mammography underuse (Casey, Call, K and Klinger, 2001; Rettig, Nelson, and Faulk, 1994). Although preventive health care utilization has increased in recent years and relationship between rural and urban residence has been quantified in previous literature, there is relatively little information available focusing on psychological, social and behavioral factors of rural women in relation to screening mammogram.

The American Cancer Society (ACS) estimates that 182,460 new cases, and 40,480 deaths from breast cancer, will occur among women in the United

States in 2008 (ACS, 2008). Overall, the rate of screening for breast cancer in the US is gradually increasing and breast cancer mortality has declined slightly. In spite of increasing screening and decreasing mortality, the mortality rates from breast cancer remain unacceptably high. Despite technological advancement in screening for breast cancer, mammography remains as the single most cost-effective method of screening for breast cancer. If used optimally, mammography could prevent 15-30% of all deaths from breast cancer through early detection (CDC, 2000). Results from several large randomized clinical trials suggest that mammography is associated with reductions of breast cancer mortality up to 39% among the 50-69 age group women (Day, 1991). Improving understanding of psychological, socio-economic and environmental factors that may influence screening behavior is a critical element of developing programs to reduce breast cancer morbidity and mortality.

Given the limited information on factors associated with participation in breast cancer screening by rural women, this project was conducted this study to measure knowledge, perceptions and behavioral practices related to breast cancer prevention among women living in a rural community in Ohio.

METHODS

Participants

The study participants were recruited from Wood County, Ohio. According to Ohio Department of Development, Office of Strategic Research data (2006), the total Wood county population is 121,065, out of which 62,461 are women. The 40 years and older age group comprised of 25,740 women who are eligible for yearly clinical breast exam and/or mammography based on the age and family history of breast cancer. Wood County is rural and its inhabitants include 4033 (3.8%) Hispanic, 1,864 (1.6%) African American and 1,514 (1.3%) Asian and Pacific Islanders among the 121,065 population. According to the Lucas and Wood County Chapter of the American Cancer Society, cancer was the second leading cause of death in 2004.

Study Design

A survey of women age 35 and older was conducted in Wood County, OH, focusing on breast cancer perceptions, knowledge, and behaviors. The survey was conducted between March 2004 and January 2005. A sample of 500 women age 35 and older was identified from the approximate 17,000 county population of women of the same age range. 35 years and older living in the Wood County, Ohio were randomly generated by a third party vendor. A personalized cover letter, along with the questionnaire, a self-addressed and stamped envelope and an incentive in the form of a crisp, new one dollar bill were mailed. A reminder letter was sent after two weeks to those who did not respond. A second reminder post-card was sent to the non-responders after four weeks. Anonymity and confidentiality was maintained by assigning codes for each questionnaire and envelop. A total of 160 completed surveys were returned in the first wave, and 90 were returned as undelivered. Thirty surveys were returned in the second wave and 45 mails were returned as undelivered. Five surveys were eliminated from the analysis because of large numbers of missing responses leaving a final study sample of 185, which translates, into a returned rate of approximately 53%. Prior to initiating data collection, approval was attained from the Institutional Review Board (IRB).

The Questionnaire

Data were collected using a 51-item questionnaire that was developed based on the constructs of Health Belief Model. Four items each were included on perceived susceptibility, severity of breast cancer and benefits of having mammogram. Seventeen items on barriers to obtaining mammograms were also included. The barrier items were developed based on the reported barriers to screening mammogram in a comprehensive literature search. To measure knowledge about breast cancer and screening mammography seventeen items on known risk factors of breast cancer, symptoms of breast cancer, and misconception about breast cancer were included. Demographics and previous behavioral practices such as previous mammogram, clinical breast examination and regular health visits were also included. To ensure content and construct validity, questionnaire was designed based on several published literature on the perception and knowledge related to breast cancer and mammogram (Friedman, Moore, Webb, and Puryear, 1999; Michielutte,

Dignan, and Smith, 1999; McDonald, Throne, Pearson, and Adams-Campbell, 1998; Crane, Kaplan, Bastani, and Scrimshaw, 1996).

Theoretical Underpinnings

According to the Health Belief Model *Perceived Susceptibility* has been defined as individual's subjective perception of his/her risk of contracting a health condition. For cases of medically established illness, such as breast cancer, perceived susceptibility includes acceptance of the diagnosis, personal estimates of susceptibly and susceptibility to illness in general (Strecher and Rosenstock, 1997).

Perceived Severity is an Individual's feelings concerning the seriousness of contracting an illness or leaving it untreated. Perceived severity also includes the evaluation of medical and clinical consequences (death, disability, pain) and possible social consequences (work, family life and social relations) associated with a disease. Individual perceptions of personal susceptibility to specific illnesses or accidents often vary from any realistic appraisal of their statistical probability (Strecher and Rosenstock, 1997). *Perceived Benefits* is defined as the decision about a course of action taken depends on beliefs regarding the effectiveness of the various available actions in reducing the disease threat, for example having a mammogram

Perceived benefits also include non-health-related benefits. The anticipated value of taking the recommended course of action is a final consideration (Strecher and Rosenstock, 1997). *Perceived Barriers* are the potential negative aspects of a particular health action may act as impediments to undertaking the recommended behavior. Perceived barriers include the costs of taking a particular action, time, difficulty, expensive or painful.

Data Management and Statistical Analysis

Original data was entered into MS Excel and converted into SPSS and SAS data format using Database Management System (DBMS). Data cleaning, coding and recoding was done before data analyses were done. Both elementary and inferential analyses were done using univariate and multivariate methods using SPSS 11.0 and SAS 9.1 version.

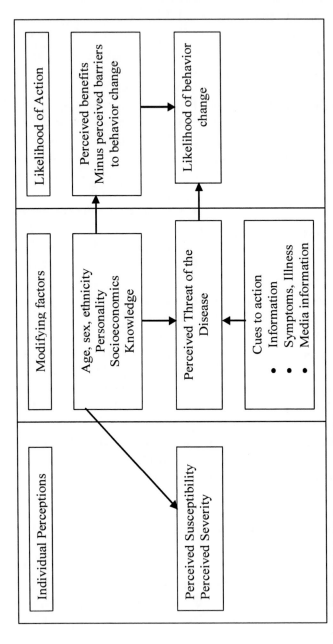

Figure 1. Health Belief Model Components and Linkages.

RESULTS

Table 1. Sociodemographic Characteristics s of the Study Respondents

	N (N= 185)	%
Age		
<40	9	5.0
40-49	58	31.4
50-59	44	23.8
60-69	30	16.0
70 and above	44	23.8
Race		
White	176	95.2
African American	5	2.7
Asian and PI	1	0.5
Hispanic	2	1.1
Other	1	0.5
Educational attainment		
< High school	9	4.9
High school grad.	56	30.4
Some College or technical school	50	27.2
College Grad.	33	17.9
> Grad. Or professional	36	19.6
Marital status		
Married	37	20.0
Single	31	16.8
Separated	3	1.6
Divorced	63	34.0
Widowed	51	27.6
Employment status		
Working full-time	94	51.4
Working part-time	11	6.0
Retired	52	28.4
Never worked	16	8.7
Not working now	10	5.5
Income level		
< $ 10,000	18	10.8
$ 10,000-$ 19,999	34	20.5
$ 20,000-$ 29,999	26	15.7
$ 30,000-$ 39,000	27	16.3
$ 40,000-$ 49,000	18	10.8
> $ 50,000	43	25.9
Insurance status		
Yes	169	91.8
No	15	8.2

The demographic characteristics of the study respondents are summarized in Table 1. The study population was all female with a mean age 38.23 years (SD=9.19). Almost all of the participants were white (95%) and all non-whites were African American. Fifty eight percent reported high school and/or some college, and another eighteen percent were college graduates. Fifty one percent were working full-time, 28% were retired, almost 11% reported annual incomes below $10,000. Twenty five percent had income level more than or equal to $50,000. Regarding health insurance, 8.2% reported not having any health insurance, 23.1% had private health insurance, 38.5% had HMO, 28% had Medicare and 11% had other types of health insurance.

Prior breast cancer screening behavior, health care utilization behavior and availability of health insurance were examined. Over 80% of the respondents reported ever having a mammogram, and of those, 76.4% had the mammogram within the past 12 months and 23.6 had a mammogram 2 years ago. The remaining respondents (14%) reporting never having had a mammogram. For clinical breast examination, 76.4% reported having had a clinical breast examination; 83.5% within the past year and 16.5% within the past 2 years. Over 90% of the respondents reported having regular health care visits; 98.1% within the past year, 1.3% between 1 and 2 years ago, and only 0.6% more than 2 years ago. Age-specific screening and health care utilization has been summarized in table 2.

Breast Cancer Knowledge

Breast cancer and screening related knowledge was assessed using 17 true-false items The items asked about early signs and symptoms of breast cancer, breast cancer risk factors, misconception about breast cancer and screening, and general knowledge of management of breast cancer. Only 1.08% women had correct answers on all items. The mean number of items answered correctly among the study population was 13 (SD=1.99). Overall the knowledge on risk factors of breast cancer was low and misconception about breast cancer was prevalent. Almost 35% women believed that being hit in the breast may cause a woman to get breast cancer later in life. About 47% women knew swelling in the breast as possible sign of breast cancer. Seventy four percent women did not think that breast cancer is more common in 65-year-old women than in 40-year-old women. About one third of the women did not know that one out of every nine women in the United Stats would develop breast cancer by the age of 85. About 41% women believed that fibrocystic breast disease (breast lumps that are not cancer) increase a woman's risk of breast cancer, and 34% women did not know breast cancer is the most common cancer in women

Table 2. Age-Specific Screening History and Health Care Utilization

Age (years)					Percentage of respondents			
	MM*Ever	MM 1 year ago	CBE MM*Ever	CBE 1 year ago	HCV	HCV 1 years ago
<40	22.2	100.0	100.0	100.0	88.9	100.0
40-49	82.8	76.3	93.1	85.1	96.6	100.0
50-59	90.9	77.4	79.6	88.0	93.2	97.5
60-69	93.3	78.3	93.3	71.4	86.7	100.0
=> 70	93.2	73.5	68.3	80.0	83.7	100.0

* Significantly different, $P < 0.05$, by χ^2 analysis

Table 3. Perceived susceptibility, Severity and Perceived Benefit Constructs

	Agree	Disagree	χ^2	P
Perceived Susceptibility				
My chances of getting breast cancer in next few years is great	39.01	60.99	8.79	0.003
Your chances of getting breast cancer in relation to average women is higher	25.82	74.18	42.55	0.001
I feel I will get breast cancer sometime during my life	21.67	78.33	57.8	<0.001
I believe all women are equally likely to develop breast cancer	32.61	67.39	22.26	<0.001
Perceived Severity				
If I had breast cancer, I would be worried and depressed	87.03	12.97	101.45	<0.001
If I had breast cancer, I would have to have my breast taken off by surgery	27.72	72.28	36.54	<0.001
If I had breast cancer, it would cause me to die	12.43	87.57	104.44	<0.001
Perceived Benefits				
I believe breast cancer can be cured easily	29.89	70.11	29.76	<0.001
If I get a mammogram and nothing is found, I would not worry about breast cancer				
If I get a mammogram and nothing is found, I would find peace of mind.	44.57	55.43	2.17	0.14
	82.61	17.39	78.26	<0.001
Regular mammogram will help finding breast lumps early and can help save my breast	93.51	6.49	140.1	<0.001
Having a regular mammogram would help my doctor save my life.	92.43	7.57	133.23	<0.001

Breast Cancer Perceptions

Perceived Susceptibility: A significant differences in perceptions of susceptibility were found. In four questions on susceptibility majority of the women disagreed- developing breast cancer in few years (61%), chance higher compared to other women (74%), and life-time risk (78%) with the p value 0.003, 0.001 and <0.001 respectively (Table 3).

Perceived Severity: Most of the women responded that they considered breast cancer as a serious disease because it will cause them worried and depressed (87%), however they disagreed on the question on surgery (72%) and breast cancer as cause of death (88%) with the p value <0.001.

Perceived Benefits of mammograms: Nearly all of the respondents reported substantial perceived benefits of mammograms and early detection. Almost 93% reported believing that regular mammograms will help finding breast lumps and help save their lives. Over 80% agreed that if nothing is found in mammography, it would bring peace of mind. However, 70% women disagreed that breast cancer can be cured easily. Almost equal number of women split up with the thought that if nothing was found in mammogram they would not worry about breast cancer (agree= 45% and disagree=55%, p=0.14).

Perceived Barriers to getting mammograms: About half (52%) of the respondents felt that gender of the provider is a barriers to mammograms, and 52% indicated that they preferred to be examined by a female physician. Thirty one percent women considered not having enough money as a barrier. However, 86% women agreed on the statement that even if mammograms are expensive, if doctors suggested that they should get it they would get it (p=0.001).

In this study the reliability of the questionnaire was assessed by item correlation. Both raw and standardized Cronbach Alpha value was over 80% (α = 0.80).

Logistic Regression

A logistic regression analysis was done to examine combinations of factors associated with regular screening mammography behavior. Previous mammogram within a year (yes versus no) was regressed with age, race, educational attainment, employment status, household income, marital status, perceptions of susceptibility, severity of breast cancer, benefits and barriers related to mammograms, recent health care visit, and clinical breast examination in the past year. Perceptions were measured in Likert scale. We created an average score on perception scale of all questions dealing with specific perception. For example, four separate questions were asked for perceived susceptibility. In the logistic regression average score of these four questions was used as a continuous variable. Both univariate and multivariate regression analyses were carried out and results are summarized in table 5.

Table 4: Perceived Barriers to Screening Mammograms

Perceived Barriers	Agree	Disagree	χ^2	P
I don't want to know if I have breast cancer or not.	5.43	94.57	146.17	0.001
Not having enough money would keep me from having a mammogram.	31.15	68.85	26.01	<0.001
I do not know where a woman can go to get a regular mammogram.	5.43	94.57	146.17	0.001
I think having a regular mammogram is too embarrassing.	8.65	91.35	126.5	<0.001
I think having a regular mammogram takes too much time.	4.32	95.68	154.38	<0.001
I would not have regular mammograms because it is likely to be painful	6.56	93.44	138.15	<0.001
Even if mammograms are expensive, if my doctor told me I should get one I would get it.	85.87	14.13	94.69	<0.001
I have trouble with transportation and that would keep me from having regular mammograms.	9.78	90.22	119.04	<0.001
I have other problems more important than having a regular mammogram.	14.13	85.87	94.70	<0.001
I think the people who give the mammograms are not careful.	3.83	96.17	156.07	<0.001
I do not have anyone to take care of my kids while I go to have mammogram.	3.14	96.86	139.63	<0.001
I would not agree to have a regular mammogram, as I do not trust mammograms.	4.32	95.68	154.39	<0.001
If I find I have breast cancer, people will treat me differently, so I don't want to have mammogram.	8.11	91.89	129.86	<0.001
I would not go for a regular mammogram, as I dislike being examined by a male physician.	3.24	96.76	161.78	<0.001
I would not go for a regular mammogram, as the result may not be kept confidential.	4.35	96.65	153.39	<0.001
I never heard or read anything encouraging having regular mammogram.	4.40	95.60	151.41	<0.001
I will prefer to have my breast examined by a female physician rather than by a male physician.	51.91	48.09	0.26	0.68

According to the univariate analysis employment status was important to getting mammograms. Women who had never been employed or who were currently unemployed were 61% less likely to have a yearly mammogram than those working part-time or fulltime (Crude OR=0.39, CI=0.16-0.97). Unmarried women were 57% less likely to have a yearly mammogram compared to married women (Crude OR=0.43, CI=0.16-1.1). Perceived barriers appeared to be a significant predictor of regular mammogram both in univariate and in adjusted model. Women were 96% less likely to have yearly mammogram for one unit increase in barrier scale (Crude OR=0.04, CI=0.01-0.14). Recent health care visit was also a significant predictor both in univariate and multivariate analyses. Women who did not visit for heath care within a year were 83% less likely to have a yearly mammogram (Crude OR=0.17, CI=0.05-0.61). Other variables were not statically significant in univariate analysis.

After controlling for all other variables perceived barriers, recent health care visit and clinical breast examination in a year appeared to be significant predictors of regular screening behavior. Women were 98% less likely to have yearly mammogram for one unit increase in barrier scale (Adjusted OR=0.02, CI=0.00-0.09).

Table 5. Crude and Adjusted Odds Ratios for Factors Associated with Screening Behavior

Factors	Crude OR	95% CI	Adjusted OR	95% CI
Age				
40-49	1.00		1.00	
<40	0.13	0.02-1.06	0.17	0.01-2.25
50-59	1.20	0.55-2.63	0.83	0.25-2.76
60-69	1.50	0.61-3.67	1.46	0.24-8.81
>=70	1.32	0.60-2.89	0.86	0.08-9.75
Race/Ethnicity				
White	1.00		1.00	
Non-White	0.44	0.11-1.80	0.09	0.01-1.52
Education				
< High school graduate	1.00		1.00	
High school graduate	1.00	0.26-3.84	3.35	0.29-38.60
Some college and technical	0.85	0.22-3.31	1.78	0.14-22.78
College and Professional	1.46	0.39-5.53	4.80	0.37-62.74

Table 5. (Continued)

Factors	Crude OR	95% CI	Adjusted OR	95% CI
Employment Status				
Full or part-time working	1.00		1.00	
Retired	1.40	0.71-2.76	1.23	0.16-9.53
Never worked or not working now	0.39	0.16-0.97*	0.34	0.06-1.87
Household Income				
< $10,000	1.00		1.00	
$10,000-$19,999	1.31	0.52-3.35		
$20,000-$29,999	2.10	0.76-5.84	3.62	0.67-19.63
$30,000-$39,999	1.41	0.52-3.83	1.31	0.29-6.00
$40,000-$49,999	1.31	0.42-4.01	0.77	0.11-5.26
>=$50,000	1.82	0.75-4.43		
Marital Status				
Married	1.00		1.00	
Divorced	0.75	0.33-1.71	0.56	0.14-2.31
Single	0.43	0.16-1.1*	0.48	0.10-2.41
Widowed	0.89	0.38-2.12	2.67	0.46-15.64
Separated	0.34	0.03-4.10	2.88	0.14-58.00
Perceptions				
Perceived Susceptibility	1.79	0.79-4.09	2.01	0.71-5.66
Perceived Severity	0.54	0.22-1.28	0.53	0.18-1.59
Perceived Benefits	1.55	0.39-6.13	2.60	0.36-18.91
Perceived Barriers	0.04	0.01-0.14*	0.02	0.03-0.09*
Recent Health Care Visit				
Yes	1.00			
No	0.17	0.05-0.61*	0.13	0.02-1.00*
Clinical Breast Examination in a Year				
Yes	1.00			
No	0.38	0.14-1.04	0.23	0.05-0.99*

Note. OR = Odds ratio; CI = Confidence interval; * = statistically significant.

Women who did not visit for heath care within a year were 87% less likely to have a yearly mammogram, though the significance level was at borderline (Adjusted OR=0.13, CI=0.02-1.00). Women who did not have clinical breast examination in a year were 77% less likely to have a yearly mammogram compared to those who had clinical breast examination in a year (Adjusted OR=0.23, CI=0.05-0.99). We examined the goodness of fit of this model by Hosmer and Lemeshow Goodness of Fit test which indicates model's goodness of fit was acceptable (Chi-sq=11.19, p=0.19).

DISCUSSION

The study population was selected from a rural community of Ohio from a randomly generated database provided by a third party vendor, which provides a basis for generalized conclusion; however, a large number of returned mails due to wrong addresses may have restricted the generalizability and lead to a selection bias. In this study population a small group of women (n=9) were less than 40 years of age. We have included them in the analysis since there was no significant difference excluding them from the analysis. The age-specific screening history and health care utilization suggests that the study population had more than state average screening rate 61.4% (CDC, BRFSS 2006) in all age groups, 76.3%, 77.4%, 78.3% and 73.5% in 40-49, 50-59, 60-69 and =>70 years respectively. Clinical breast examination a year ago was also similar except for the age group 60-69, who are below the state average (71.4% versus 78.7%).

Though perceived susceptibility did not appear to be a significant predictor in this study population, however, the perception on susceptibility is noteworthy. In all four questions majority of the women did not perceive themselves as susceptible to develop breast cancer. Women in this study had high severity perception and they also perceived mammography as beneficial for cancer prevention. However, 55% women did not think that if nothing was found in screening mammogram they would not worry about breast cancer. Approximately 72% women did not think that if they were diagnosed with breast cancer surgical removal of breast will be done. In one hand these women were concern about being worried and depressed if they were diagnosed with breast cancer, on the other hand, they do not believe that surgery will be done as treatment; fear or denial might have played a role in this situation. About fear or denial in other population similar findings were found (Rahman, Dignan, and Shelton, 2003; Rahman, Mohamed, and Dignan, 2003; Rahman, Dignan, and Shelton, 2005).

Recent health care visit appeared to be a significant predictor associated with yearly mammography behavior both in univariate and multivariate analysis, though after adjusting for all other variables it was at the borderline significance level. In previous studies, women who visited a gynecologist as usual care physician had highest rate of mammography (Finison, Wellins, Wennberg, and Lucas, 1999). Physician's recommendation or motivational suggestion from health care professional was found to be effective in promoting mammography (Fox, Klos, and Tsou, 1988; Fox, Murata, and Stein, 1991; Burns, Freund, Ash, Shwartz, and Antab, 1995). In this study 86% women agreed that irrespective of expenses they would have had a mammogram if it was recommended by their physicians. Clinical breast examination in a year also appeared as significant factor associated with yearly screening mammogram. This finding is consistent with the previous studies where regular health care visit or other screening behavior influenced screening mammography.

This study has several limitations. Though the questionnaire was sent to a total of 500 randomly selected women, a large number of returned mails due to wrong address may have caused selection bias. We followed the empirical findings on survey cash incentives between no cash versus one dollar incentives (James, and Bolstein,1992; Lesser, Dillman, Lorenz, Carlson, and Brown, 1999) where they found 12 percent point increase return, and only an additional two to seven percent point increase for five and ten dollar incentives. In our study most of the women who returned the completed survey also returned the one dollar bill. Another limitation is we do not have any objective assessment of breast cancer screening behavior. However, several studies have found high validity of self-reported breast cancer screening behavior and considered self-report as useful information (Paskett et al., 1996; Zapka et al., 1996). Apart from these limitations the study findings clearly show that the rural population are lacking in knowledge about breast cancer, screening mammograms and have low perceived susceptibility of breast cancer. Future behavioral interventions should focus on novel approaches to counteract the perceived barriers to increase unitization of screening and to prevent breast cancer in this population.

REFERENCES

American Cancer Society. *Cancer Facts and Figures 2008.* Atlanta-American Cancer Society: 2008.

Burns, R., Freund, K., Ash, A., Shwartz, M., and Antab, L. (1995). Who gets Repeat screening Mammography: The Role of the Physician. *Journal of General Internal Medicine, 10*, 520-522.

Casey, M. M., Call, K.T., and Klinger, J.M. (2001). Are rural residents less likely to obtain recommended preventive health care services? *American Journal of Preventive Medicine, 21(3),* 182-188.

Center for Disease Control and Prevention (2000).

Center for Disease Control and Prevention, BRFSS, 2006

Crane, L.A., Kaplan, C.P., Bastani, R., and Scrimshaw, S.C.M. (1996). Determinants of adherence among health department patients referred for a mammogram. *Women and Health, 24 (2),* 43-64.

Day, N. E. (1991). Screening for breast cancer. *Br Med Bull, 47,* 400-15.

Finison, K.S., Wellins, C.A., Wennberg, D.E., and Lucas, F.L. (1999). Screening mammography rates by specialty of the usual care physician. *Eff. Clin. Pract; 2,* 120-5.

Fox, S., Klos, D., and Tsou, C. (1988). Under use of screening mammography by family physicians. *Radiology, 166,* 431-433.

Fox, S., Murata, P., and Stein, J. (1991). The impact of physician compliance on screening mammography of older women. *Archives of Int. Medicine, 151,* 50-56.

Friedman, L.C., Moore, A., Webb, J. A, and Puryear, L. J. (1999). Breast cancer screening among ethnically diverse low-income women in a general hospital psychiatry clinic. *General Hospital Psychiatry*, 21, 374-381.

Hochbaum, G. (1958). *Public Participation in Medical Screening Programs: A sociopsychological study.* Washington, DC: Government Printing Office.

James, J.M. and Bolstein, R. (1992). Large monetary incentives and their effect on mail survey response rates. *Public Opinion Quaterly, 56,* 442-453.

Lesser, V., Dillman, D.A., Lorenz, F.O., Carlson, J., and Brown, T.L. (1999). The influence of financial incentives on mail questionnaire response rates. Paper presented at the meeting of the Rural Sociological Society, Portland, OR.

Liff, J., Chow, W., and Greenburg, R. (1991). Rural-urban differences in stage at diagnosis: possible relationship to cancer screening. *Cancer; 67*, 1454-9.

Monroe, A., Ricketts, T., and Savitz, L. (1992). Cancer in rural versus urban population: a review. *Journal of Rural Health; 8*, 212-220.

Michielutte, R., Dignan, M., and Smith, B. (1999). Psychosocial factors associated with the use of breast cancer screening by women age 60 years or over. *Health Education and Behavior, 26*, 625-647.

McDonald, P.A.G., Throne D.D., Pearson J.C., and Adams-Campbell, L. L., (1999). Perceptions and knowledge of breast cancer among African-American women residing in public housing. *Ethnicity and Disease, 9*, 82-93.

Office of Strategic Research, Ohio Department of Development (2006). Population and Housing Data.

Paskett E.D., Tatum C.M., Mack D.W., Hoen, H., Case, L.D., and Velez, R. (1996). Validation of self-reported breast and cervical cancer screening tests among low-income minority women. *Cancer Epidemiol Biomarkers Prev, 5*, 721-726.

Rahman, S.M.M., Dignan, M.B., and Shelton, B.J. (2003). Factors influencing adherence to guidelines for screening mammography among women aged 40 years and older, *Ethnicity and Disease, 13(4),* 477-484.

Rahman, S.M.M., Mohamed, I., Dignan M.B. (2003). Assessment of Perceptions Related to Breast Cancer Prevention and Behavioral Practices in Medically Underserved Women, *The Journal of Multicultural Nursing and Health, 9(3)*, 30-39.

Rahman, S.M.M., Dignan, M.B., Shelton B.J. (2005). A theory-based prediction model for adherence to guidelines for screening mammography among women age 40 and older. *International Journal of Cancer Prevention, 2* (3), 169-79.

Rettig, B., Nelson, N., and Faulk, R. (1994). Breast cancer screening recent trends in the use of mammography in Nebraska. *Nebr Med J, 136*,13.

Rosenstock, I. (1974). Historical origin of Health Belief Model. *Health Education Monographs, 2,* 328-335.

SAS version 9.1 (2006), SAS Institute Inc.

SPSS version 11.0 (2005), SPSS Inc.

Stearns, S.C., Bernard S.L., Fasick S.B, Schwartz, R., Konrad, T. R., Ory, M. G., et al. (2000). The economic implications of self-care: the effect of life-style, functional adaptations, and medical self-care among national sample of Medicare beneficiaries. *American Journal of Public Health, 90(10),* 1608-1612.

Stretcher V.J. and Rosenstock I.M. (1997) The Health Belief Model. In *Health Behavior and Health Education: Theory, Research, and Practice* (Glanz K., Lewis F.M. and Rimer B.K., eds), Jossey-Bass, San Francisco, CA, pp. 41–59.

Zapka, J.G., Bigelow, C., Hurley, T., Ford, L.D., Egelhofer, J., Cloud, W.M., et al. (1996). Mammography use among socioeconomically diverse women: the accuracy of self-report. *Am J Pubic Health. 86,*1016-1021.

Zhang, P., Tao, G., and Irwin, K.L. (2000). Utilization of preventive medical services in the United States: a comparison between rural and urban populations. *Journal of Rural Health; 16(4),* 349-56.

This study was funded by Research Incentive Grant (RIG) at the Bowling Green State University, OH, USA.

In: Breast Cancer Screening and Prevention   ISBN 978-1-61209-288-1
Editor: Jonathan D. Pegg   © 2011 Nova Science Publishers, Inc.

Chapter 4

ACCESS TO MAMMOGRAPHY FACILITIES AND DETECTION OF BREAST CANCER BY SCREENING MAMMOGRAPHY: A GIS APPROACH

Selina Rahman[*1,2], *James H. Price*[2],
Mark Dignan[4], *Saleh Rahman*[5], *Peter S. Lindquist*[3] *and Timothy R. Jordan*[2]

[1] Environmental Sciences Institute, Florida A and M University
[2] Department of Health and Human Services, University of Toledo
[3] Department of Geography and Planning, University of Toledo
[4] Prevention Research Center, University of Kentuckey
[5] Institute of Public Health, Florida AandM University

* Corresponding Author: MBBS, PhD, MPH, Research Associate, Adjunct Faculty, Institute of Public Health, Florida A and M University, FSH Science Research Center, 209-A, 1515 South ML King Street, Tallahassee, FL 32307, Phone: 850 980 2864, Fax: 850 599 8830, Email: Selina.rahman@famu.edu

ABSTRACT

Objectives: The objective of the study was to examine the association between access to mammography facilities and utilization of screening mammography in an urban population.

Methods: Data on female breast cancer cases were obtained from an extensive mammography surveillance project. Distance to mammography facilities was measured by using GIS, which was followed by measuring geographical access to mammography facilities using Floating Catchment Area (FCA) Method (considering all available facilities within an arbitrary radius from the woman's residence by using Arc GIS 9.0 software).

Results: Of 2,024 women, 91.4% were Caucasian; age ranged from 25 to 98 years; most (95%) were non-Hispanic in origin. Logistic regression found age, family history, hormone replacement therapy, physician recommendation, and breast cancer stage at diagnosis to be significant predictors of having had a previous mammogram. Women having higher access to mammography facilities were less likely to have had a previous mammogram compared to women who had low access, considering all the facilities within 10 miles (OR=0.41, CI=0.22-0.76), 30 miles (OR=0.52, CI=0.29-0.91) and 40 miles (OR=0.51, CI=0.28-0.92) radiuses. *Conclusions:* Physical distance to mammography facilities does not necessarily predict utilization of mammogram and greater access does not assure greater utilizations, due to constraints imposed by socio economic and cultural barriers. Future studies should focus on measuring access to mammography facilities capturing a broader dimension of access considering qualitative aspect of facilities, as well as other travel impedances.

Keywords: Mammography, GIS, access, distance, breast cancer.

INTRODUCTION

Breast cancer is one of the leading causes of death among women in the United States. The American Cancer Society estimated that 178,480 new cases and 40,460 deaths from breast cancer occurred among women in the United

States in 2007 (American Cancer Society [ACS], 2007). Due to a lack of primary prevention of breast cancer, breast cancer mortality and morbidity reduction depends on secondary prevention, chiefly through screening mammography. Several randomized trials as well as population-based screening evaluations have indicated that early detection of breast cancer through screening mammography improves treatment options, the likelihood of successful treatment, and improved survival (William, Holladay, and Sheikh 2003; Taber et al., 2003; Humphrey, Helfand, Chan, and Woolf, 2002; Duffy, Tabar, and Chen, 2002). A rise in mammography utilization is suggested by the observed trends (1987-1999) of an increase in breast cancer incidence confined to early stage breast cancer (Howe, et al., 2001; Edwards, et al., 2002; Blanchard, et al. 2004). A significant and substantial reduction in female breast cancer mortality has been observed in recent years because of screening mammography (Smith, et al., 2003; Duffy et al., 2006). However, the mortality rate from breast cancer is still too high, even though screening rates have increased and mortality decreased somewhat. The Healthy People 2010 target is 22.3 deaths per 100,000 women, but according to the American Cancer Society data the death rate is 26 per 100,000 women in 2007 (ACS, 2007).

Several researchers have explored barriers to obtaining mammograms, including the physical distance to mammography facilities and other barriers (Ann, Ronald, Raymond, and Gilligan, 2001; Jilda, Hyndman, and Holman, 2000a; Jilda, Hyndman, and Holman, 2000b). Understanding the geographical and social connections between the utilization of mammography and the locations of mammography facilities is critically important for developing effective programs to reduce breast cancer mortality. Health Education Promotion programs designed to increase mammography screening and produce subsequent reduction in breast cancer mortality may have opportunities to improve their effectiveness if they are able take barriers such as geographic distance to screening services into consideration. Health care decisions are strongly influenced by the type and quality of services available in the local area and the distance, time, cost, and ease of traveling to reach those services (Goodman, Fisher, Stukel, and Chang, 1997; Haynes, Bentham, Lovett, and Gale, 1999; Joseph and Phillips, 1984; Croner, Sperling, and Broome, 1996; Fortney, Rost, and Warren, 2003). The term 'spatial accessibility' is gaining more and more attention in the health care geography literature (Khan and Bhardwaj, 1994; Luo, 2004; Luo and Wang, 2003), which is a combination of dimensions of accessibility (travel impedance between patients and service points, that is measured in units of distance or travel time), and availability (refers to the number of local service locations from which a patient can choose). In this study, we focused on measuring access to mammogram facility by using GIS, considering both accessibility and availability dimensions. We also examined whether access to mammography facilities and other demographic variables influence utilization of mammography.

METHODS

Data Collection

The data for this study were obtained from the Colorado Mammography Project (CMAP). CMAP was a National Cancer Institute funded project that was in operation from 1994-2004. CMAP was one member of a seven-site consortium, and obtained data on mammograms from approximately half of all mammography facilities in the six-county Denver metropolitan area of Colorado. For this study, information on mammograms for women from 1999-2001 was analyzed. The CMAP database included demographic data (age, race/ethnicity, education, and insurance status), data on mammogram results, previous mammogram history, family history, use of hormone replacement therapy, physician recommendation, and the zip codes of women's residences. Addresses of mammography facilities participating in CMAP were obtained for this study from the Colorado Department of Public Health and Environment. There were 46 facilities on the list that were operating during the time period (1999-2001) and were considered as the possible facilities that women might use to obtain a mammogram.

Calculation of Access to Mammography Facility

We used the "Floating catchment area" (FCA) method by Luo and Wang (2004) to calculate access, that considered all available facilities within an arbitrary radius around a woman's address. Forty-six mammography facilities were geocoded using the ArcGIS System and placed in a separate file. Zip code centroids were obtained from a Zip code polygon file and compared to the database of patients. All Zip code centroids that had no patients from the sample were discarded, and then the numbers of patients were summed for each Zip code centroid and placed in a separate file. Mammography facility points and Zip code centroid points were connected to the regional street and highway network. Point-to-Point mileages were computed in a separate shortest path utility embedded within the GIS. The mileages were outputted in the form of a distance matrix. The distance matrix between Zip code centroids and mammography facilities was then imported into an Excel spreadsheet. Minimum distance that a woman would be willing to travel to get to a mammogram was considered 10, 20, 30, 40, or, 50 miles and following operations were performed for each of these arbitrary radius. For each specified radius, the number of women among all Zip codes within the specified radius was summed for each of the 46 mammography facilities identified within the study area. Then the inverse of these sums were computed to calculate the availability of that facility. Now, for each woman's Zip code within a specified radius, the availability for all facilities was summed to obtain the FCA index, representing her access to mammogram facility. Finally, indices for five different arbitrary radii 10, 20, 30, 40, and 50 miles were computed to calculate access to mammography facility.

Statistical Analysis to Examine Relationship between the Variables

To further explore the association between the variables, logistic regressionwas performed. The dependent variable entered into the logistic model was whether the woman has had a previous mammogram or not (coded as yes=1 and No=0). Women who had a previous record of mammogram in the CMAP database or answered, "yes" on their patient information form when asked about their previous mammogram history at their index examination were considered as having had a previous mammogram (Figure 1 displays the distribution of the study population that did not have a previous mammogram in the six county areas).

A series of categorical variables were created and entered into the logistic model such as, age, race/ethnicity, education, insurance status, family history, hormone replacement therapy, physician recommendation, and breast cancer stage at diagnosis along with access to mammography facilities. Among the independent variables, the 'physician recommendation' variable was divided into two broad categories: 'diagnostic' that included all the diagnostic procedures (such as, biopsy, needle localization, and ultrasound) and 'evaluative' that included the rest of the categories, such as, follow up, physical examination, surgical consultation etc. Breast cancer stage at diagnosis was also condensed into two categories: non-advanced breast cancer stage at diagnosis included carcinoma *in situ*, and localized tumors, which are malignant and invasive but confined to the organ of origin; and advanced stage of breast cancer at diagnosis included regional neoplasm that have extended beyond the organ of origin into surrounding tissues, involving regional lymph nodes, or both, and distant tumors that have spread to remote parts of the body from the primary site.

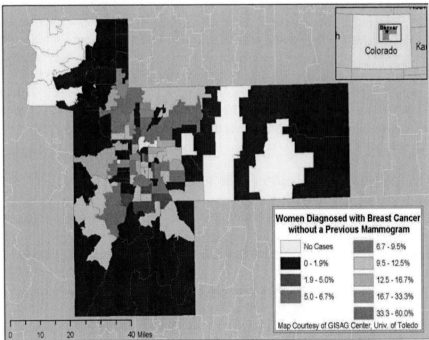

Figure 1. Distribution of Population Who did not have had a Previous Mammogram (by Zip Code).

With the access ratio for five different radii (such as, 10 miles, 20 miles, 30 miles, 40 miles, and 50 miles) five different logistic regression models were developed. Both univariate and multivariate analyses were conducted and on the basis of analysis of maximum likelihood estimates, significant interaction terms were identified and there was no significant interaction between the variables.

RESULTS

Demographic Characteristics

The data from the Colorado Cancer Registry included 2042 individuals diagnosed with breast cancer during the period of 1999 to 2001. Descriptive statistics for the study population are summarized in Table 1.

The breast cancer cases ranged in age from 25 to 98 years with 30% being 50-59 years of age and nearly all were Caucasian (91%). Twenty one percent reported having Medicaid and/or Medicare and 78% also had private insurance.

Among those with data on family history, 17% had a positive family history of breast cancer. Among those with data on hormone replacement therapy, 42% were on hormone replacement therapy at the time of the initial mammogram. Nearly all (91%) of the women in the database had a previous mammogram.

Table 2 presents the odds ratios for the factors influencing having had a previous mammogram. Access to mammography facilities was negatively associated with having had a previous mammogram in the adjusted model developed for 10 miles, 30 miles, and 40 miles radius. Women who had greater access to mammography facilities were 59% less likely and women who had medium access to such facilities were 58% less likely respectively of having had a previous mammogram, compared to women who had low access to mammography facilities; and these findings were significant in both the crude and adjusted models for the 10 miles radius measure.

For the 30 miles radius access measure, women who had high access to mammography facilities was 48% less likely of having had a previous mammogram when compared to women who had less access to mammography facilities (OR = 0.52, 95% CI = 0.29-0.91).

The odds of having had a previous mammogram for women who had high access to mammography facilities were 0.51(95% CI= 0.28-0.92) times compared to women who had less access to mammography facilities and these findings were significant for both the crude and adjusted models developed for the 40 miles radius access measure. The 50 miles radius access measure finding was not statistically significant in any model.

Table 1. Characteristics of the Study Population

Factors	Number (N=2042)	Percentage (%)
Age		
Below 40 years	121	6
40-49	503	24
50-59	609	30
60-69	364	18
70 years and above	445	22
Race/Ethnicity		
White	1811	91
Black	45	2
Asian	17	<1
American Indians and others	5	<1
Hispanic	104	5
Ethnicity		
Hispanic	104	5
Non Hispanic	1898	95
Education		
Less than High School Graduate	46	6
High School Graduate	198	26
Some College	251	32
College, or Post Graduate	280	36
Insurance Status		
Medicaid and/or Medicare	392	21
No Insurance	15	<1
Other (Private insurance, managed care and others)	1417	78
Stage of Breast Cancer		
In situ	320	16
Localized	1080	56
Regional	498	26
Direct	32	2
Previous mammogram		
Yes	1560	91
No	155	9
Family History		
Yes	190	17
No	953	83
Hormone replacement therapy		
Yes	440	42
No	608	58
Physician Recommendation		
Diagnostic	497	46
Evaluative	585	54

Note. Totals do not add to 2042 because of missing values.

Percentage calculated based on the non-missing values.

Table 2. OR for Factors Predicting Women who had a Previous Mammogram

Factors	Crude OR	95% CI	Adjusted OR	95% CI
Age Group				
Below 40 years	0.13	0.07-0.22*	0.11	0.06-0.22*
40-49	1.00		1.00	
50-59	3.24	1.81-5.80*	1.63	0.80-3.32
60-69	2.79	1.44-5.40*	1.72	0.77-3.90
70 years and above	0.73	0.47-1.14	1.02	0.50-2.09
Race/Ethnicity				
White	1.00		1.00	
Black	0.45	0.18-1.10	0.68	0.20-2.19
Asian	1.57	0.21-11.89	2.75	0.21-35.65
Hispanic	0.37	0.21-0.66*	0.51	0.06-4.69
Ethnicity				
Hispanic	1.00		1.00	
Non Hispanic	2.03	1.17-3.52*	1.55	0.19-12.82
Education				
Less than High School Graduate	1.00		1.00	
High School Graduate	0.33	0.20-0.54*	0.66	0.34-1.26
Some College	0.32	0.21-0.51*	0.65	0.36-1.19
College, or Post Graduate	0.38	0.24-0.60*	0.82	0.44-1.51
Insurance Status				
Medicaid and/or Medicare	0.38	0.19-0.75*	0.48	0.20-1.17
No insurance	1.00		1.00	
Other (Private insurance, managed care and others)	0.64	0.34-1.22	0.95	0.43-2.13
Family History				
Yes	1.00		1.00	
No	0.18	0.11-0.28*	0.37	0.19-0.69*
Hormone replacement therapy				
Yes	1.00		1.00	
No	0.09	0.06-0.14*	0.15	0.08-0.27*
Physician Recommendation				
Diagnostic	1.00		1.00	
Evaluative	1.23	0.85-1.77	2.00	1.24-3.23*
Breast cancer stage at diagnosis				
Non-advance stage	1.00		1.00	
Advance stage	0.58	0.41-0.83*	0.69	0.43-1.10

Table 2. (Continued)

Factors		Crude OR	95% CI	Adjusted OR	95% CI
Access to mammogram facilities					
Within 10 miles radius	High access	0.46	0.27-0.77*	0.41	0.22-0.76*
	Medium access	0.42	0.25-0.71*	0.42	0.23-0.76*
	Low access	1.00		1.00	
Within 20 miles radius	High access	0.60	0.38-0.96*	0.58	0.34-1.00
	Medium access	0.81	0.49-1.35	0.72	0.39-1.31
	Low access	1.00		1.00	
Within 30 miles radius	High access	0.68	0.42-1.10	0.52	0.29-0.91*
	Medium access	0.67	0.41-1.09	0.85	0.49-1.49
	Low access	1.00		1.00	
Within 40 miles radius	High access	0.58	0.35-0.97*	0.51	0.28-0.92*
	Medium access	0.79	0.47-1.32	0.68	0.37-1.25
	Low access	1.00		1.00	
Within 50 miles radius	High access	0.91	0.50-1.63	0.82	0.41-1.61
	Medium access	0.81	0.46-1.44	0.78	0.40-1.51
	Low access	1.00		1.00	

Note. OR = Odds ratio; CI = Confidence interval; * = statistically significant.
(Adjusted Odds ratio for all the independent variables are taken from the logistic model for 30 mile radius)

In Table 2, after adjustment for all other variables, women in the age group below 40 years were negatively associated with having had a previous mammogram when compared to women in the age group 40-49 years, which was statistically significant (adjusted OR = 0.11, 95% CI = 0.06-0.22). After adjustment for other variables, neither race nor ethnicity remained significantly associated with having had a previous mammogram when compared with White women. Women's educational attainment level and insurance status were not statistically significantly associated with having had a previous mammogram in the adjusted model. Not having a family history of breast cancer appeared as a negative predictor of having had a previous mammogram in the adjusted model, as it had in the univariate model, and remained statistically significant (adjusted OR = 0.37, 95% CI = 0.19-0.69). The odds of having had a previous mammogram for women who did not have a family history of breast cancer were about one-third as likely as women who had a positive family history of breast cancer. Hormone replacement therapy remained negatively associated with having had a previous mammogram after controlling for all other variables in the adjusted model (adjusted OR = 0.15, 95% CI = 0.08-0.27) and the finding was statistically significant. In the adjusted model after controlling for all other variables, the evaluative recommendation by physicians was found to be a significant predictor of having had a previous mammogram (OR = 2.00, 95% CI = 1.24-3.23).

DISCUSSION

The gravity model, a combined measure of accessibility and availability was used to evaluate the potential spatial interaction between any woman's location and all alternative mammography facilities within a reasonable distance. The relationship of geographical access and utilization of mammogram is noteworthy. In Denver metropolitan area most of mammography facilities are located close to the downtown where accessibility is higher. Women diagnosed with breast cancer without a previous mammogram also higher in this area (Figure 1). In another study we found women diagnosed with advanced stage of breast cancer are also higher in these areas (Rahman, et al., 2007). Several issues contribute in determining which mammography facility to be used to get a mammogram, or more specifically, why a woman would not use the nearest mammography facility or just one facility to obtain her mammograms. Factors such as the type of health insurance and their policies regarding reimbursement may have determined which mammography facility a woman must use to get a mammogram. A common physician practice is to recommend their patients to a specific mammography facility. Some women may prefer to go to a mammography facility that is closer to their work place rather than from their residence. Moreover, it is crucial to specify one mammogram facility that the woman used to measure the straight-line distance from her residence. Typically for a diagnosis of breast cancer a woman will have one or two mammograms and then an ultrasound, which will be followed by a biopsy and all of these examinations usually do not occur within the same clinic or on the same day.

Both access and distance are equally important in considering barriers to overcome for screening mammogram and diagnostic testings for breast cancer. Being hindered in either way would likely result in a later stage of breast cancer at diagnosis. Taking into account all the above issues it seems more appropriate that we measure access to mammogram facility considering all the available facilities within an arbitrary radius, rather than the distance from the woman's residence to nearest facility or one specific facility.

Again, in the literature the arbitrary radius is usually considered as 30 miles for FCA method; however most of these studies are about primary care rather than preventive care. Assuming that the minimum distance a woman would be willing to travel to get a preventive service, such as, mammogram would be different, access ratio for several different radii (10, 20, 30, 40, and 50 miles) were measured and compared. While comparing access measures of different arbitrary radiuses in the FCA method, as the radius increased from 10 miles to 50 miles, the standard deviation of access measures decreased and also the range from minimum to maximum decreased (Table 3).

This indicates that the access measure with a higher radius had less variance, which led to stronger spatial smoothing, which is a manifestation of MAUP (modifiable areal unit problem). Access scores tended to increase with increasing radius, as one would have more access if she were permitted or capable of traveling further. As the radius increased from 10 miles to 50 miles, the population with high access also increased (Figure 2, Figure 3 and Figure 4).

Table 3. Comparison of Accessibility Measures

Radius	Total number	Minimum	Maximum	Mean	Std. Deviation
10 Mile	1745	.0000000	.1075926	.0263610	.0261128
20 Mile	1745	.0000000	.0768412	.0263610	.0136416
30 Mile	1745	.0000000	.0536146	.0263610	.0084047
40 Mile	1745	.0000000	.0377056	.0263610	.0056572
50 Mile	1745	.0011524	.0314764	.0263610	.0042359

N= 2042.
Frequency missing 297.

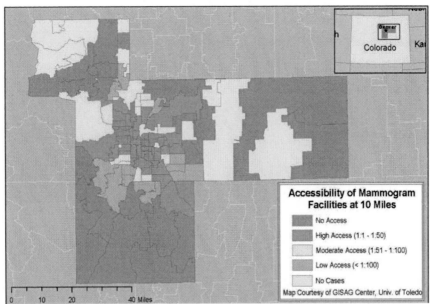
Figure 2. Accessibility to Mammogram Facilities within 10 Miles Radius (by Zip Code).

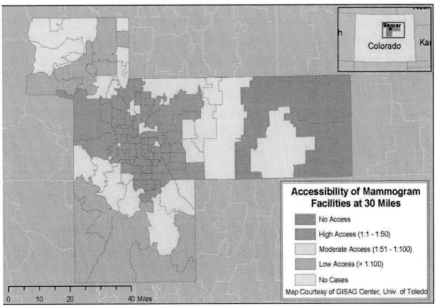
Figure 3. Accessibility to Mammogram Facilities within 30 Miles Radius (by Zip Code).

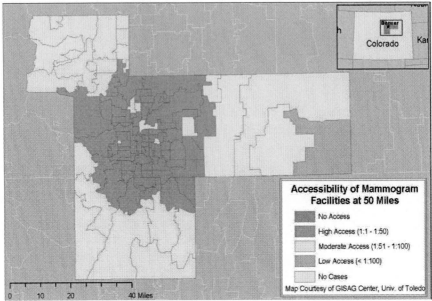

Figure 4. Accessibility to Mammogram Facilities within 50 Miles Radius (by Zip Code).

However, if we look at the mean access measure for the population, it remains the same for all the measures with different radiuses (Table 3) as because increasing radius does not necessarily mean increasing access. Access depends on the distribution of supply of and demand for mammograms. In the method of calculating access to mammography facilities in the current study, the availability of the facility was considered only by the total number of women sharing that facility, which meant that all the mammography facilities were viewed as having equal capacity. When the radius increased, the number of women within that arbitrary radius increased as well, which acted to decrease the ultimate access to a mammography facility as more women shared that facility. To overcome this limitation, future research is needed that will consider the qualitative aspects of the mammography facilities, such as, the size, number of staff members, amount of equipment and other details that might have affected the capacity of a facility.

Several other limitations that were related to the access measure of the current study are as follows: First, the population data were geocoded by using women's Zip codes as exact addresses were not available because of a requirement to maintain confidentiality. By using Zip codes, women were assigned to an area rather than assigned to a single point. This technique might have decreased the level of precision for the measure of access to mammography facility. Second, the current study was limited to only six county areas. A known limitation of the FCA method in measuring access is that people within a catchment area have equal access to all providers within that same catchment area, and all providers beyond the radius of the catchment area are inaccessible, regardless of any differences in distances (Luo, 2004; Luo and Wang, 2004;). Finally, absence of individual level data on income or socio-economic status and missing data on health insurance, education, hormone replacement therapy, family history, physician recommendation and previous mammogram were also a major limitation of the current study.

ACKNOWLEDGMENT

Dr. Fahui Wang, Department of Geography, Northern Illinois University.

REFERENCES

American Cancer Society: *Cancer Facts and Figure ures 2003-2004*. Atlanta, American Cancer Society, Inc, 2005.

Ann, B.N., Ronald, T.K., Raymond, G.H., and Gilligan, M.A. (2001). Relationship of distance from a radiotherapy facility and initial breast cancer treatment. *Journal of National Cancer Institute. 93(17)*, 1344-1346.

Blanchard, K., Colbert, J.A., Puri, D., Weissman, J., Moy, B., Kopans, D.B. et al. (2004). Mammographic screening: Patterns of use and estimated impact on breast carcinoma survival. *Cancer, 101*, 495-507.

Croner, C.M., Sperling, J., and Broome, F. R. (1996). Geographic information systems (GIS): New perspectives in understanding human health and environmental relationships. *Statistics in Medicine, 15*, 1961-1977.

Duffy, S., Taber, L., Chen, H.H., Smith, A., Holmberg, L., Jonsson, H., et al., (2006). Reduction in Breast Cancer Mortality from Organized Service Screening with Mammography: 1. Further Confirmation with Extended Data. *Cancer Epidemiol Biomarkers Prev, 15(1)*, 45–51.

Duffy, S., Taber, L., and Chen, H.H. (2002). The impact of organized mammographic service screening on breast cancer mortality in seven Swedish counties. *Cancer, 95*, 458-469.

Edwards, B.K., Howe, H.L., Ries, L.A.G., Thun, M.J., Rosenberg, H.M., Yancik, R., et al. (2002). Annual report to the Nation on the status of cancer, 1973-1999, featuring implications of age and aging on US cancer burden. *Cancer, 94,* 2766-2792.

Fortney, J., Rost, K., and Warren, J. (2003). Comparing alternative methods of measuring geographic access to health services. *Health Services and Outcomes Research Methodology.* 1(2): 173-184.

Goodman, D., Fisher, E., Stukel, T., and Chang, C. (1997). The distance to community medical care and the likelihood of hospitalization: Is closer always better? *Am. J. Public Health, 87,*144–50.

Haynes, R., Bentham, G., Lovett, A., and Gale, S. (1999). Effects of distances to hospital and GP surgery on hospital inpatient episodes controlling for needs and provision. *Soc. Sci. Med, 49,* 425–433.

Howe, H. L., Wingo, P. A., Thun, M. J., Ries, L. A. G., Rosenberg, H. M., Feigal, E.G. et al. (2001). Annual report to the nation on the status of cancer (1973 through 1998), features cancers with recent increasing trends. *J. Natl. Cancer Inst, 93,* 824-842.

Humphrey, L.L., Helfand, M., Chan, B.K., Woolf, S.H. (2002). Breast cancer screening: a summary of the evidence for the U.S. Preventive Services Task Force. *Ann. Intern. Med., 137(5),* 347-360.

Jilda, C.G., Hyndman, C. D'Arcy, and Holman, J. (2000a). Differential effects on socioeconomic groups of modelling the location of mammography screening clinics using geographic information systems. *Australian and New Zealand Journal of Public Health, 24(3),* 281-286.

Jilda, C.G., Hyndman, C. D'Arcy, and Holman, J. (2000b). Effect of distance and social disadvantage on the response to invitations to attend mammography screening. *J. Med. Screen, 7,* 141-145.

Joseph, A., and Phillips, D. (1984). *Accessibility and Utilization: Geographical Perspectives on Health Care Delivery.* New York: Harper and Row.

Khan, A. A. and Bhardwaj, S. M. (1994). Access to health care: A conceptual framework and its relevance to health care planning. *Evaluation and the Health Professions. 17(1)* : 60-76.

Luo, W. (2004). Using a GIS-based floating catchment method to assess areas with shortage of physicians. *Health and Place, 10,* 1-11.

Luo, W., and Wang, F. (2003). Measures of spatial accessibility to health care in a GIS environment: synthesis and a case study in the Chicago region. *Environment and Planning B: Planning and Design, 30,* 865-884.

Rahman, S., Price, J. M., Dignan, M., Rahman, S. M., Lindquist, P. S., and Jordan, T. M. (2007). Access to mammography facilities and breast cancer stage at diagnosis: A GIS approach. Paper accepted for oral presentation at the AACE Annual Meeting 2007 (Oct 11-13): Cancer Education in Minority and Underserved Populations. UAB Comprehensive Cancer Center, Alabama.

Smith, R.A., Saslow, D., Sawyer, K.A., Burke, W., Costanza, M.E., Evans, W.P., et al.(2003). American Cancer Society guidelines for breast cancer screening: Update 2003. *CA Cancer J. Clin., 53(3),* 141-169.

Tabar, L., Yen, M.F., Vitak, B., Chen, H.H., Smith, R.A., and Duffy, S.W. (2003). Mammography service screening and mortality in breast cancer patients: 20-year follow-up before and after introduction of screening. *Lancet, 361(9367),* 1405-1410.

Williams, W.H., Holladay, D.A., and Sheikh, A.A., et al. (2003). Practical impact of screening mammography: Analysis of Pathological factors and treatment utilization for women undergoing breast conservation therapy at a large radiation therapy center. *Proc. Am. Soc. Clin. Oncol. , 22,* 87-95.

In: Breast Cancer Screening and Prevention   ISBN 978-1-61209-288-1
Editor: Jonathan D. Pegg   © 2011 Nova Science Publishers, Inc.

Chapter 5

ACCESS TO MAMMOGRAPHY FACILITIES AND BREAST CANCER STAGE AT DIAGNOSIS: DOES GEOGRAPHIC DISTANCE PREDICT?

Saleh M. M. Rahman[*1], *Selina Rahman*[2],
Mark B. Dignan[3] *and Peter S. Lindquist*[4]

[1]Behavioral Sciences and Health Education, Institute of Public Health,
Florida A and M University College of Pharmacy and Pharmaceutical
Sciences, 209-A FSH Science Research Center, Tallahassee, FL 32307
[2]Environmental Sciences Institute, Florida A and M University
[3]Prevention Research Center, University of Kentuckey4 Department of
Health and Human Services, University of Toledo
[4]Department of Geography and Planning, University of Toledo

ABSTRACT

This study examined the association between access to mammography facilities and breast cancer stage at diagnosis in an urban

[*] Corresponding author: Ph: 850-599-8840; Fax: 850-599-8830; E-mail: E-mail:
saleh.rahman@famu.edu

population. Data on female breast cancer cases were obtained from an extensive mammography surveillance project. The Floating Catchment Area Method, considering all available facilities within an arbitrary radius from woman's residence, was used to assess access to mammography facilities. Results showed that odds of breast cancer being diagnosed at an advanced stage were higher for women who had greater access compared to women who had lower access to mammogram facilities. Greater access did not assure breast cancer to be diagnosed at less advanced stage due to constraints imposed by socio economic and cultural barriers. Future studies should measure access to mammography facilities capturing a broader dimension of access.

INTRODUCTION

Breast cancer is one of the leading causes of death among women in the United States. An estimated 178,480 new cases and 40,460 deaths from breast cancer are expected to occur among women in the United States in 2007 (ACS, 2007). Due to a lack of primary prevention of breast cancer, breast cancer mortality and morbidity reduction depends on secondary prevention, chiefly through screening mammography. Several randomized trials as well as population-based screening evaluations have indicated that early detection of breast cancer through screening mammography improves treatment options, the likelihood of successful treatment, and improved survival (William, Holladay, Sheikh, et al., 2003; Taber, Yen, Vitak, et al., 2003; Humphrey, Helfand, Chan, and Woolf, 2002; Duffy, Tabar, and Chen, 2002). Moreover, several studies found significant down staging of breast cancers associated with mammography screening (Freedman, Anderson, Goldstein, Hanlon, et al., 2003; Vacek, Geller, Weaver, and Foster, 2002; Ernster, Ballard-Barbash, Barlow, et al., 2002; Wu, Weissfeld, Weinberg, and Kuller, 1999; McCarthy, Burns, Freund, et al., 2000; Solin, Schultz, Legorreta, and Goodman, 1995). Breast cancer stage and size down staging in women with a history of mammography screening was also found to be associated with breast conserving treatment (Freedman, Anderson, Goldstein, Hanlon, et al., 2003). This is consistent with the observed trend for the increasing use of breast conserving treatment in the United States, particularly among women with stage I breast carcinomas (Stewart, Bland, McGinnis, Morrow, and Eyre, 2000; Solin, Legorreta, Schultz, et al., 1994; Roberts, Alexander, Anderson, et al., 1990; Andersson, Aspegren, Janzon, et al., 1988). Research also shows a significant and substantial reduction in female breast cancer mortality in recent years associated with use of screening mammography (Smith, et al., 2003; Duffy et al., 2006). However, the mortality rate from breast cancer is still too high, even though screening rates have increased and mortality decreased somewhat. The Healthy People 2010 target is 22.3 deaths per 100,000 women, but according to the American Cancer Society data the death rate is 26 per 100,000 women in 2007 (American Cancer Society, 2007).

Several studies have explored barriers to obtaining mammograms, including distance to mammography facilities (Ann, Ronald, Raymond, Gilligan, 2001; Jilda, Hyndman, Holman, 2000; Jilda, Hyndman, Holman, 2000). Understanding the geographic and health service factors is critically important for developing effective programs to reduce breast cancer mortality. Health education/promotion programs designed to increase mammography screening and produce subsequent reduction in breast cancer mortality may have opportunities to improve their effectiveness if they are better able to include consideration of barriers such as geographic distance to screening services in planning. Health care decisions are strongly influenced by the type and quality of services available in the local area and the distance, time, cost, and ease of traveling to reach those services (Goodman, Fisher, Stukel, and Chang, 1997; Haynes, Bentham, Lovett, and Gale, 1999; Joseph and Phillips, 1984; Croner, 1996; Fortney, Rost and Warren, 2003).

The term 'spatial accessibility' is gaining attention in the health care geography literature (Khan and Bhardwaj, 1994; Luo, 2004; Luo and Wang, 2003). Spatial accessibility is a combination of dimensions of accessibility (travel impedance between clients and service points, which is measured in units of distance or travel time) and availability (refers to the number of local service locations from which a client can choose). In this study, we focused on measuring access to mammogram facility by using GIS, considering both accessibility and availability dimensions. We also examined whether access to mammography facilities and other demographic variables influence breast cancer stage at diagnosis.

METHODS

The data for current study were obtained from the Colorado Mammography Project (CMAP). CMAP was a National Cancer Institute funded project that was in operation from 1994-2004. CMAP was one member of a seven-site consortium, and obtained data on mammograms from approximately half of all mammography facilities in the six-county Denver metropolitan area of Colorado. For the present study, information on breast cancer cases from 1999-2001 was analyzed. Breast cancers for the present analyses included invasive cancers and ductal carcinoma *in situ* (DCIS) but did not include localized carcinoma *in situ* (LCIS). All cases were diagnosed based on the diagnostic criteria recommended by the American Medical Association and the Colorado Cancer Registry. The CMAP database included demographic data (age, race/ethnicity, education, and insurance status), data on mammogram results, whether there was a previous mammogram, family history, use of hormone replacement therapy, physician recommendation, and the zip codes of women's residences. Addresses of mammography facilities participating in CMAP were obtained for this study from the Colorado Department of Public Health and Environment. There were 46 facilities on the list that were operating during the time period (1999-2001) and were considered as the possible facilities that women might use to obtain a mammogram.

Calculation of Distance and Access to Mammography Facility

We used the "Floating catchment area" (FCA) method by Luo and Wang (2004) to calculate distance and access. We considered all available facilities within an arbitrary radius around a woman's address, rather than just measuring the straight-line distance from the woman's residence to nearest facility or one specific facility. The FCA method requires a spatially distributed population count at census tract or block group level and the number of providers in the study area as the inputs for the analysis (Luo and Wang, 2003, Luo, 2004). Distance was calculated by road network analysis. Shortest paths were computed on the highway network using a version of Moore's Algorithm embedded within the ArcGIS software package. Once the travel distance was calculated from woman's residence Zip code to mammography facilities, the FCA method was applied for calculating accessibility. Steps taken in the computation were as follows:

1. The 46 mammography facilities were geocoded using the ArcGIS System and placed in a separate file.

2. Zip code centroids were obtained from a Zip code polygon file and compared to the database of patients. All Zip code centroids that had no patients from the sample were discarded, leaving only those centroids that had patients. The numbers of patients were summed for each Zip code centroid and placed in a separate file.

3. Mammography facility points and Zip code centroid points were connected to the regional street and highway network. Point-to-Point mileages were computed in a separate shortest path utility embedded within the GIS. The mileages were outputted in the form of a distance matrix.

4. The distance matrix between Zip code centroids and mammography facilities was imported into an Excel Spreadsheet. The following operations were performed among radii of 10, 20, 30, 40 and 50 miles. For each specified radius, the number of women among all Zip codes within the specified radius was summed for each of the 46 mammography facilities identified within the study area. Then the inverse of these sums were computed and summed for each zip code to obtain the FCA index inputted into the regression model. Finally, indices for 10, 20, 30, 40, and 50 miles were computed and placed in a table on another worksheet within an Excel spreadsheet file.

Statistical Analysis to Examine Relationship between the Variables

To further explore the association between the variables, logistic regression analysis was performed. The dependent variable entered into the logistic model was 'breast cancer stage at diagnosis' (coded as advanced = 1, non-advanced = 0); non-advanced breast cancer stage at diagnosis included carcinoma *in situ*, and Stage 1 (localized tumors); all other Stages were coded as advanced. A series of categorical variables were created and entered into the logistic model such as, age, race/ethnicity, education, insurance status, family history, hormone replacement therapy, physician recommendation, and previous mammogram along with access to mammography facilities (coded as high access=1, medium access=2, and low access=3). Among the independent variables, the 'Physician recommendation' variable was divided into two broad categories: 'diagnostic' that included all the diagnostic procedures (such as, biopsy, needle localization, and ultrasound) and 'evaluative' that included the rest of the categories, such as, follow up, physical examination, surgical consultation etc. Women who had a previous record of mammogram in the CMAP database or answered, "yes" on their patient information form when asked about their previous mammogram history at their index examination were considered as having had a previous mammogram. With the access ratio for five different radii (such as, 10 miles, 20 miles, 30 miles, 40 miles, and 50 miles) five different logistic regression models were developed. Both univariate and multivariate analyses were conducted and on the basis of analysis of maximum likelihood estimates, significant interaction terms were identified and there was no significant interaction between the variables.

RESULTS

Demographic Characteristics

Data on 2042 breast cancer cases diagnosed during the period of 1999 to 2001 were included in the analyses. Descriptive statistics for the study population are summarized in Table 1. The breast cancer cases ranged in age from 25 to 98 years with 30% being 50-59 years of age and nearly all were Caucasian (91%). Twenty one percent reported having Medicaid and/or Medicare and 78% also had private insurance.

Table 1. Characteristics of the Study Population

Factors	Number (N=2042)	Percentage (%)
Age		
Below 40 years	121	6
40-49	503	24
50-59	609	30
60-69	364	18
70 years and above	445	22
Race/Ethnicity		
White	1811	91
Black	45	2
Asian	17	<1
American Indians and others	5	<1
Hispanic	104	5
Ethnicity		
Hispanic	104	5
Non Hispanic	1898	95

Table 1. (Continued)

Education		
Less than High School Graduate	46	6
High School Graduate	198	26
Some College	251	32
College, or Post Graduate	280	36
Insurance Status		
Medicaid and/or Medicare	392	21
No Insurance	15	<1
Other (Private insurance, managed care and others)	1417	78
Stage of Breast Cancer		
In situ	320	16
Localized	1080	56
Regional	498	26
Direct	32	2
Previous mammogram		
Yes	1560	91
No	155	9
Family History		
Yes	190	17
No	953	83
Hormone replacement therapy		
Yes	440	42
No	608	58
Physician Recommendation		
Diagnostic	497	46
Evaluative	585	54

Note. Totals do not add to 2042 because of missing values. Percentage calculated based on the non-missing values.

Among those with data on family history, 17% had a positive family history of breast cancer. Among the non-advanced stage of breast cancer cases, 16% had carcinoma *in- situ,* 56% had localized breast cancer; and advanced stage included 26% regional stage of breast cancer, and 2% distant metastases (Figure 1 displays distribution of breast cancer stages at diagnosis by Zip Codes).

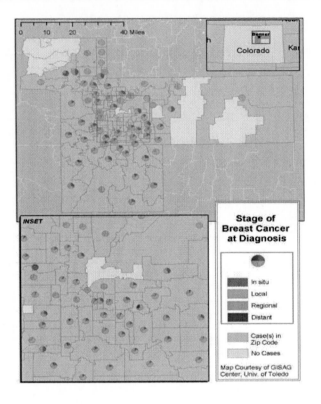

Figure 1. Distribution of Breast Cancer Stage at Diagnosis (by Zip Code).

Distance figures were calculated first as a straight-line distance between centroids of two Zip codes (woman's residence Zip code and mammography facility Zip code); mean distance from the woman's residence Zip code to a mammography facility Zip code was 13 miles with a standard deviation of 41 miles and a range of less than one mile to 638 miles. Access ratio is then calculated by FCA method for each woman for several different radii such as, 10 miles, 20 miles, 30 miles, 40 miles, and 50 miles. Table 2 and Figure 2, Figure 3 and Figure 4 depict a comparison of access measures of different arbitrary radiuses. As the radius in the FCA method increased from 10 miles to 50 miles, the standard deviation of access measures decreased and also the range from minimum to maximum decreased, though the mean access measure for the population remained the same for all the measures with different radii.

Accessibility of Mammogram Facilities at 10 Miles (by Zip Code)

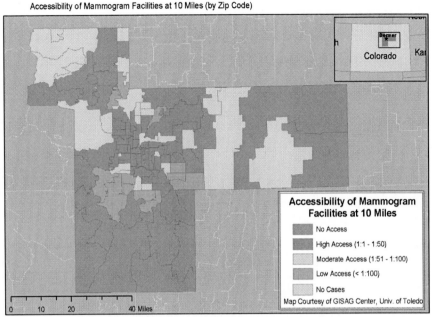

Figure 2. Accessibility to Mammogram Facilities within 10 Miles Radius (by Zip Code).

Table-3 presents crude and adjusted odds ratios for the factors influencing breast cancer stage at diagnosis using access measures. Adjusted odds ratios for all the independent variables are reported from the logistic regression model for the 50-miles radius model. After adjustment for all other variables, the odds of breast cancer being diagnosed at an advanced stage for women who had medium access compared to women who had low access was 1.53 times, when the minimum distance a woman would be willing to travel was considered as 50 miles (adjusted OR = 1.53, 95% CI = 1.08-2.15).

Accessibility of Mammogram Facilities at 30 Miles (by Zip Code)

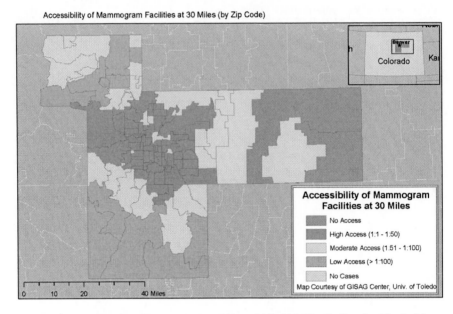

Figure 3. Accessibility to Mammogram Facilities within 30 Miles Radius (by Zip Code).

Table 2. Comparison of Accessibility Measures

Radius	Total number	Minimum	Maximum	Mean	Std. Deviation
10 Mile	1745	.0000000	.1075926	.0263610	.0261128
20 Mile	1745	.0000000	.0768412	.0263610	.0136416
30 Mile	1745	.0000000	.0536146	.0263610	.0084047
40 Mile	1745	.0000000	.0377056	.0263610	.0056572
50 Mile	1745	.0011524	.0314764	.0263610	.0042359

N= 2042. Frequency missing 297.

Table 3. Crude and Adjusted Odds Ratios for Factors Predicting Advanced Stage Breast Cancer at Diagnosis Using Access Measure

Factors	Crude OR	95% CI	Adjusted OR	95% CI
Age Group				
Below 40 years	1.43	0.94-2.18	1.55	0.98-2.44
40-49	1.00		1.00	
50-59	0.89	0.69-1.16	0.95	0.71-1.28
60-69	0.81	0.59-1.09	0.81	0.56-1.51
70 years and above	0.65	0.48-0.88*	0.63	0.41-0.95*

Race/Ethnicity						
White		1.00		1.00		
Black		1.06	0.54-2.08	0.83	0.40-1.71	
Asian		1.51	0.63-3.62	1.53	0.62-3.80	
Hispanic		0.87	0.54-1.40	1.97	0.61-6.39	
Ethnicity						
Hispanic		1.00		1.00		
Non Hispanic		1.32	0.86-2.01	2.22	0.76-6.50	
Education						
Less than High School Graduate		1.00		1.00		
High School Graduate		0.75	0.52-1.09	0.73	0.50-1.15	
Some College		1.58	1.18-2.11*	1.52	1.04-2.21*	
College, or Post Graduate		1.05	0.78-1.41	1.00	0.69-1.48	
Insurance Status						
Medicaid and/or Medicare		0.78	0.53-1.13	0.94	0.58-1.50	
No insurance		1.00		1.00		
Other (Private insurance, managed care and others)		1.04	0.76-1.42	0.94	0.66-1.36	
Previous mammogram						
Yes		0.69	0.55-0.87*	0.72	0.54-0.96*	
No		1.00		1.00		
Family History						
Yes		1.00		1.00		
No		1.11	0.91-1.36	1.19	0.89-1.60	
Hormone replacement therapy						
Yes		1.00		1.00		
No		1.20	0.97-1.49	1.06	0.79-1.43	
Physician Recommendation						
Diagnostic		1.00		1.00		
Evaluative		0.81	0.64-1.01	0.77	0.58-1.02	
Within 10 miles radius	High access	0.88	0.68-1.15	0.94	0.71-1.23	
	Medium access	0.91	0.70-1.19	0.98	0.74-1.28	
	Low access	1.00		1.00		
Within 20 miles radius	High access	1.01	0.78-1.31	1.09	0.83-1.43	
	Medium access	1.02	0.78-1.34	1.10	0.83-1.46	
	Low access	1.00		1.00		
Access to mammogram facilities						
Within 30 miles radius	High access	1.07	0.82-1.40	1.15	0.87-1.50	
	Medium access	0.89	0.69-1.17	0.92	0.69-1.21	
	Low access	1.00		1.00		
Within 40 miles radius	High access	1.10	0.83-1.47	1.23	0.91-1.65	
	Medium access	1.09	0.83-1.43	1.21	0.91-1.60	
	Low access	1.00		1.00		

Table 3. (Continued)

Within 50 miles	High access	1.23	0.87-1.73	1.38	0.97-1.97
radius	Medium access	1.40	1.00-1.95*	1.53	1.08-2.15*
	Low access	1.00		1.00	

Note. OR = Odds ratio; CI = Confidence interval; * = statistically significant.
(Adjusted Odds ratio for all the independent variables are taken from the logistic model for 50 miles radius).

Accessibility of Mammogram Facilities at 50 Miles (by Zip Code)

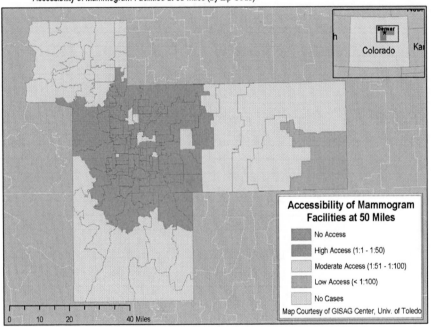

Figure 4. Accessibility to Mammogram Facilities within 50 Miles Radius (by Zip Code).

After adjustment for all other variables, the age group 70 years and older was negatively associated with advanced stage of breast cancer at diagnosis, which was statistically significant (OR = 0.63, 95% CI = 0.41-0.95). This finding implies that the oldest women were less likely to be diagnosed with breast cancer at an advanced stage compared to younger women. Women who have had a previous mammogram were 28% less likely to have their breast cancer diagnosed at an advanced stage compared to women who did not have a previous mammogram in the adjusted model and the finding was statistically significant (adjusted OR = 0.72, 95% CI= 0.54-0.96). Education was also found to be a significant predictor of breast cancer stage at diagnosis. In the adjusted model, the odds of having breast cancer diagnosed at an advanced stage for women having some college degree were 1.52 times as likely as women who had less than a high school degree and the finding was statistically significant (adjusted OR = 1.52, 95% CI= 1.04-2.21). Race/ethnicity was not a significant predictor for breast cancer stage at diagnosis after adjustment for all other variables. Family history and hormone replacement therapy were positively associated with breast cancer stage at diagnosis, but was not statistically significantly different in the adjusted model. When entered into the adjusted model after adjustment for other variables, physician recommendation was found to be negatively associated with breast cancer stage at diagnosis, but the finding was not statistically significant (adjusted OR = 0.77, 95% CI = 0.58-1.02).

DISCUSSION

The current study used a combined measure of accessibility and availability to evaluate the potential spatial interaction between any woman's residence and all alternative mammography facilities within a reasonable distance. This is a unique approach to study access to mammography facilities in a situation for women especially in an urban setting. Because several issues contribute in determining which mammography facility to be used to get a mammogram, or more specifically, why a woman would not use the nearest mammography facility or just one facility to obtain her mammograms. Factors such as the type of health insurance and their policies regarding reimbursement may have determined which mammography facility a woman must use to get a mammogram. A common physician practice is to recommend their patients to a specific mammography facility. Some women may prefer to go to a mammography facility that is closer to their work place rather than from their residence. Moreover, it is crucial to specify one mammogram facility that was used by a woman to diagnose breast cancer. Typically the diagnosis of breast cancer occurs through step by step procedures such as mammograms, ultrasound, and biopsy, and all of these procedures usually do not occur within the same clinic or on the same day. Both access and distance are equally important in considering barriers to overcome for mammogram and diagnostic testing as both access and distance may be associated with later stage of cancer at diagnosis. Taking into account all the above issues it seems more appropriate that we measure access to mammogram facility considering all the available facilities within an arbitrary radius, rather than the distance from the woman's residence to nearest facility or one specific facility. Access scores were measured in several different radii and as the radius increased from 10 miles to 50 miles, the population with high access also increased. Nevertheless, if we look at the mean access measure for the population, it remains the same for all the measures with different radiuses (Table 2) as because increasing radius does not necessarily mean increasing access. Access depends on the distribution of supply of and demand for mammograms. In the method of calculating access to mammography facilities in the current study, the availability of the facility was considered only by the total number of women sharing that facility, which meant that all the mammography facilities were viewed as having equal capacity. When the radius increased, the number of women within that arbitrary radius increased as well, which acted to decrease the ultimate access to a mammography facility as more women shared that facility. To overcome this limitation, future research is needed that will consider the qualitative aspects of the mammography facilities, such as, the size, number of staff members, amount of equipment and other details that might have affected the capacity of a facility.

Several other limitations that were related to the access measure of the current study are as follows: First, the population data were geocoded by using women's Zip codes as exact addresses were not available because of a requirement to maintain confidentiality. By using Zip codes, women were assigned to an area rather than assigned to a single point. This technique might have decreased the level of precision for the measure of access to mammography facility. Second, the current study was limited to only six county areas. A known limitation of the FCA method in measuring access is that people within a catchment area have equal access to all providers within that same catchment area, and all providers beyond the radius of the catchment area are inaccessible, regardless of any differences in distances (Luo and Wang, 2003; Luo, 2004). Finally, absence of individual level data on income or socio-economic status and missing data on health insurance, education, hormone replacement therapy, family history, physician recommendation and previous mammogram were also a major limitation of the current study.

REFERENCES

American Cancer Society: Cancer Facts and Figures 2005-2006. Atlanta, American Cancer Society, Inc, 2007.

Andersson I, Aspegren K, Janzon L et al, 1988. Mammographic screening and mortality from breast cancer: The Malmo mammographic screening trial. *Br. Med. J.* 297: 943-948.

Ann BN, Ronald TK, Raymond GH, Gilligan MA. (2001). Relationship of distance from a radiotherapy facility and initial breast cancer treatment. *Journal of National Cancer Institute. 93(17),* 1344-1346.

Blanchard K, Colbert JA, Puri D, Weissman J, Moy B et al. (2004). Mammographic screening: Patterns of use and estimated impact on breast carcinoma survival. *Cancer, 101,* 495-507.

Croner C.M. et al. (1996). Geographic information systems (GIS): new perspectives in understanding human health and environmental relationships. *Statistics in Medicine, 15,* 1961-1977.

Duffy S, Taber L, Chen HH, et al. (2002). The impact of organized mammographic service screening on breast cancer mortality in seven Swedish counties. *Cancer, 95,* 458-469.

Duffy S, Taber L, Chen HH, Smith A., Holmberg L., et al., (2006). Reduction in Breast Cancer Mortality from Organized Service Screening with Mammography: 1. Further Confirmation with Extended Data. *Cancer Epidemiol. Biomarkers Prev., 15(1),* 45–51

Edwards BK, Howe HL, Ries LAG, Thun MJ, Rosenberg HM, Yancik R, Wingo PA, Jemal A, Feigal EG. (2002). Annual report to the Nation on the status of cancer, 1973-1999, featuring implications of age and aging on US cancer burden. *Cancer, 94,* 2766-2792.

Ernster VL, Ballard-Barbash R, Barlow WE, et al., (2002). Detection of ductal carcinoma in situ in women undergoing screening mammography. *J. Natl. Cancer Inst., 94,* 1546-1554.Fotheringham, A. S., and Rogerson, P. A. (Eds.). (1994). Spatial analysis and GIS. London: Taylor and Francis.

Fortney J., Rost K. and Warren J. (2003). Comparing alternative methods of measuring geographic access to health services. *Health Services and Outcomes Research Methodology.* 1(2): 173-184.

Freedman GM, Anderson PR, Goldstein LJ, Hanlon AL, Cianfrocca ME et al., 2003. Routine mammography is associated with earlier stage disease and greater eligibility for breast conservation in breast carcinoma patients age 40 years and older. *Cancer* 98(5): 918-925.

Fotheringham, A. S., and Rogerson, P. A. (Eds.). (1994). Spatial analysis and GIS. London: Taylor and Francis.

Goodman D, Fisher E, Stukel T, Chang C. (1997). The distance to community medical care and the likelihood of hospitalization: Is closer always better? *Am. J. Public Health, 87,*144–50.

Haynes R, Bentham G, Lovett A, Gale S. (1999). Effects of distances to hospital and GP surgery on hospital inpatient episodes controlling for needs and provision. *Soc.Sci. Med, 49,* 425–433.

Howe HL, Wingo PA, Thun MJ, et al. (2001). Annual report to the nation on the status of cancer (1973 through 1998), features cancers with recent increasing trends. *J. Natl. Cancer Inst, 93,* 824-842.

Humphrey LL, Helfand M, Chan BK, Woolf SH. (2002). Breast cancer screening: a summary of the evidence for the U.S. Preventive Services Task Force. *Ann Intern Med, 137(5),* 347-360.Jelinski DE, Wu J (1996) The modifiable areal unit problem and implications for landscape ecology. *Landsc. Ecol.* 11:120–140.

Jelinski DE, Wu J (1996) The modifiable areal unit problem and implications for landscape ecology. Landsc Ecol 11:120–140

Jilda C.G. Hyndman, C. D'Arcy J. Holman. (2000). Differential effects on socioeconomic groups of modelling the location of mammography screening clinics using geographic information systems. *Australian and New Zealand Journal of Public Health, 24(3),* 281-286.

Jilda C.G. Hyndman, C. D'Arcy J. Holman. (2000). Effect of distance and social disadvantage on the response to invitations to attend mammography screening. *J. Med. Screen, 7,* 141-145.

Joseph A, Phillips D. (1984). *Accessibility and Utilization: Geographical Perspectives on Health Care Delivery.* New York: Harper and Row.

Luo W and Wang F. (2003). Measures of spatial accessibility to health care in a GIS environment: synthesis and a case study in the Chicago region. *Environment and Planning B: Planning and Design, 30,* 865-884.

Luo W. (2004). Using a GIS-based floating catchment method to assess areas with shortage of physicians. *Health and Place, 10,* 1-11.

Martin D, Wrigley H, Barnett S, Roderick P. (2002). Increasing the sophistication of access measurement in a rural healthcare study. *Health Place, 8,* 3–13.

McCarthy EP, Burns SB, Freund KM, et al., (2000). Mammography use, breast cancer stage at diagnosis, and survival among older women. *J. Am. Geriatr. Soc., 48,* 1226-1233

Roberts MM, Alexander FE, Anderson TJ, et al, 1990. Edinburg trial of screening for breast cancer: Mortality at seven years. *Lancet;* 335: 241-246

Smith RA, Saslow D, Sawyer KA, Burke W, Costanza ME, Evans WP, Foster RS, Hendrick E, Eyre JJ, Sener S. (2003). American Cancer Society guidelines for breast cancer screening: Update 2003. *CA Cancer J. Clin., 53(3),* 141-169.

Solin LJ, Schultz DJ, Legorreta AP , Goodman RL. 1995. Down staging of breast carcinomas associated with mammographic screening. *Breast Diseases.* 8: 45-56.

Solin LJ, Legorreta AP, Schultz DJ, et al, 1994. The importance of mammographic screening relative to the treatment of women with carcinoma of breast. Arch Intern Med; 154: 745-752.

Stewart AK, Bland KI, McGinnis LS Jr., Morrow M, Eyre HJ. (2000). Clinical highlights from the National Cancer Data Base, 2000. *CA Cancer J. Clin., 50,* 171-183.

Tabar L, Yen MF, Vitak B, Chen HH, Smith RA, Duffy SW. (2003). Mammography service screening and mortality in breast cancer patients: 20-year follow-up before and after introduction of screening. *Lancet, 361(9367),* 1405-1410.

Vacek PM, Geller BM, Weaver DL, Foster RS Jr. (2002). Increased mammography use and its impact on earlier breast cancer detection in Vermont, 1975-1999. *Cancer, 94,* 2160-2168.

Williams WH, Holladay DA, and Sheikh AA, et al (2003). Practical impact of screening mammography: Analysis of Pathological factors and treatment utilization for women undergoing breast conservation therapy at a large radiation therapy center. *Proc. Am. Soc. Clin. Onco., 22,* 87-95.

Wu Y, Weissfeld JL, Weinberg GB, Kuller LH, (1999). Screening mammography and late-stage breast cancer: a population based study

In: Breast Cancer Screening and Prevention   ISBN 978-1-61209-288-1
Editor: Jonathan D. Pegg   © 2011 Nova Science Publishers, Inc.

Chapter 6

REDUCTION IN THE RISK OF HUMAN BREAST CANCER BY SELECTIVE CYCLOOXYGENASE-2 (COX-2) INHIBITORS: FINAL RESULTS OF A CASE CONTROL STUDY

Randall E. Harris*, Joanne Beebe-Donk
and Galal A. Alshafie
The Ohio State University College of Medicine and Public Health
320 West 10th Avenue
Columbus, Ohio, USA 43210-1240

ABSTRACT

Background
    Epidemiologic and laboratory investigations suggest that non-steroidal anti-inflammatory drugs (NSAIDs) have chemopreventive effects against breast cancer due to their activity against cyclooxygenase-2 (COX-2), the rate-limiting enzyme of the prostaglandin cascade.

---

* Corresponding author: harris.44@osu.edu

Methods

We conducted a case control study of breast cancer designed to compare effects of selective and non-selective COX-2 inhibitors. A total of 611 incident breast cancer patients were ascertained from the James Cancer Hospital, Columbus, Ohio, during 2003-2004 and compared with 615 cancer free controls frequency-matched to the cases on age, race, and county of residence. Data on the past and current use of prescription and over the counter medications and breast cancer risk factors were ascertained using a standardized risk factor questionnaire. Effects of COX-2 inhibiting agents were quantified by calculating odds ratios (OR) and 95% confidence intervals.

Results

Results showed significant risk reductions for selective COX-2 inhibitors as a group (OR=0.15, 95% CI=0.08-0.28), regular aspirin (OR=0.46, 95% CI = 0.32-0.65), and ibuprofen or naproxen (0.36, 95% CI= 0.21-0.60). Intake of COX-2 inhibitors produced significant risk reductions for premenopausal women (OR=0.05), postmenopausal women (OR=0.26), women with a positive family history (OR=0.19), women with a negative family history (OR=0.14), women with estrogen receptor positive tumors (OR=0.24), women with estrogen receptor negative tumors (OR=0.05), women with HER-2/neu positive tumors (OR=0.26), and women with HER-2/neu negative tumors (OR=0.17). Acetaminophen, a compound with negligible COX-2 activity produced no significant change in the risk of breast cancer.

Conclusions

Selective COX-2 inhibitors (celecoxib and rofecoxib) were only recently approved for use in 1999, and rofecoxib (Vioxx) was withdrawn from the marketplace in 2004. Nevertheless, even in the short window of exposure to these compounds, the selective COX-2 inhibitors produced a significant (85%) reduction in the risk of breast cancer, underscoring their strong potential for breast cancer chemoprevention.

Both the magnitude and the direction of effect of selective COX-2 blockers on the risk of cardiovascular disease is the subject of controversy. Risk *increases* have been observed with use of rofecoxib and celecoxib in clinical trials that were designed to evaluate their potential for treating arthritis or reducing colonic polyp recurrence [3, 4, 5], whereas risk *decreases* have been observed in observational studies that were designed to evaluate effects of these same compounds on cardiovascular diseases [6, 7, 8]. Still other investigations suggest that COX-2 inhibitors have no effect on the risk of myocardial infarction and related cardiovascular events [9, 10].

Among American women, breast cancer is the most frequently diagnosed malignancy and second leading cause of cancer death [11]. Despite intensive efforts aimed primarily at early detection and therapy, the mortality rates of breast cancer have remained virtually constant for several decades. Innovative research efforts must therefore be redirected towards chemoprevention of the early stages of carcinogenesis. Among twenty published epidemiologic studies that focused on the association between intake of nonsteroidal anti-inflammatory drugs (NSAIDs) and the risk of human breast cancer, 13 reported statistically significant risk reductions. Meta-analysis of these data suggests that regular NSAID intake significantly reduces the risk of breast cancer [12].

Two selective COX-2 inhibitors, celecoxib (Celebrex) and rofecoxib (Vioxx), were approved for the treatment of arthritis by the United States Food and Drug Administration (FDA) in 1999. Until the recall of Vioxx in September, 2004, these two compounds plus other selective COX-2 inhibitors valdecoxib (Bextra) and meloxicam (Mobic) were widely utilized in the United States for pain relief and treatment of osteoarthritis and rheumatoid arthritis. The time period between approval of Celebrex to the recall of Vioxx provides an approximate six-year window for evaluation of exposure to such compounds by a case control approach. The current case control study was designed to test the chemopreventive value of selective COX-2 blockade against human breast cancer.

METHODS

We studied 611 cases of invasive breast cancer with histological verification based upon review of the pathology records, and 615 group-matched controls with no personal history of cancer and no current breast disease based on screening mammography. Cases were sequentially ascertained for interview at the time of their diagnosis during 2003 through September, 2004 at The Arthur G. James Cancer Hospital and Richard J. Solove Research Institute (CHRI), Columbus, Ohio. There were no refusals to participate among cases. The controls were ascertained from the mammography service of the cancer hospital during the same time period and frequency matched to the cases by five-year age interval, race, and place (county) of residence. Controls were sequentially ascertained for each matching category resulting in a stratified random sample. Among women eligible for participation, 95% completed the questionnaire.

Critical information on exposure to NSAIDs and other factors were obtained utilizing a standardized risk factor questionnaire. The questionnaires were administered in person by trained medical personnel prior to definitive surgery or treatment for the cases and at the time of screening mammography for controls. The data variables collected consisted of demographic characteristics, height, weight, menstrual and pregnancy history, family history of breast and ovarian cancer, comprehensive information on cigarette smoking, alcohol intake, pre-existing medical conditions (arthritis, chronic headache, cardiovascular conditions including hypertension, angina, ischemic attacks, stroke, and myocardial infarction, lung disease, and diabetes mellitus), and medication history including over the counter (OTC) and prescription NSAIDs, and exogenous hormones. Regarding selective COX-2 inhibitors and other NSAIDs, the use pattern (frequency, dose, and duration), and the type, (celecoxib, valdecoxib, rofecoxib, meloxicam, aspirin, ibuprofen, naproxen, indomethacin) were recorded. Data on the related analgesic, acetaminophen were collected for comparison with selective COX-2 inhibitors and other NSAIDs.

Case-control differences in means and frequencies were checked for statistical significance by t-tests and chi square tests, respectively. Effects of the selective COX-2 inhibitors as a group were quantified by estimating odds ratios and their 95% confidence intervals. Odds ratios were adjusted for age and classical breast cancer risk factors (parity, family history, body mass, menopausal status, chronic smoking, and regular alcohol intake) by logistic regression analysis [13, 14]. Adjusted estimates were obtained for specific types of compounds, e.g., over the counter NSAIDs, selective COX-2 inhibitors, and acetaminophen. Estimates for selective COX-2 inhibitors were checked for stability by conducting subgroup analyses by menopausal status, family history, and estrogen receptor and human epidermal growth factor receptor (HER-2/neu) status.

RESULTS

Pertinent characteristics of the cases and controls are given in Table 1. The cases exhibited higher frequencies of nulliparity, family history of breast or ovarian cancer, estrogen replacement therapy in postmenopausal subjects, and chronic cigarette smoking. As expected, cases and controls had similar distributions of age, race, and education.

Table 1. Characteristics of breast cancer cases and controls

Characteristic [a]	Cases (N=323)	Controls (N=649)
Age (yrs)		
<50	19%	20 %
50-65	55	52
>65	26	28
Mean (SEM)	55.8 (0.8)	55.2 (0.4)
Race		
Caucasian	91 %	89 %
All Other	9	11
Education		
< 12 yrs	12 %	12 %
12 yrs	53	55
> 12 yrs	31	33
Parity		
Nulliparous	6 %	4 %
First Pregnancy <30 yrs	83	89
First Pregnancy >30 yrs	11	7 (p<0.05)
Family History		
Positive	32 %	17 %
Negative	68	83 (p<0.01)
Body Mass		
BMI < 22	23 %	21 %
BMI 22-28	35	39
BMI > 28	42	40
Mean (SEM)	27.5 (0.9)	27.1 (0.7)
Menopausal Status		
Premenopausal	41 %	47 %
Postmenopausal	52	53
Postmenopausal ERT	38	31 (p<0.05)
Smoking		
Never smoker	35 %	32 %
Ex-smoker	38	40
Current smoker	27	28
Alcohol Intake		
None	47 %	45 %
1-2 drinks per week	36	35
> 2 drinks per week	17	20

[a] Family History: either breast or ovarian cancer among first or second degree female relatives; ERT=Estrogen Replacement Therapy for two or more years; Body Mass Index = weight (kg) / ht ^{2} (m).

Table 2 shows the comparative frequencies of the medications under study with odds ratios and 95% confidence intervals. Multivariate-adjusted estimates are presented. A significant reduction in the risk of breast cancer was observed for daily intake of selective COX-2 inhibitors for two years or more (OR=0.15, 95% CI=0.08-0.28). Observed risk reductions were consistent for the individual COX-2 inhibitors, celecoxib (OR=0.14, 95% CI=0.05-0.43) and rofecoxib (OR=0.15, 95% CI= 0.06-0.37). Significant risk reductions were also observed for the intake of two or more pills per week of aspirin (OR=0.46, 95% CI= 0.32-0.65) and ibuprofen or naproxen (OR=0.36, 95% CI=0.21-0.60). Acetaminophen, an analgesic with negligible COX-2 activity had no effect on the relative risk of breast cancer (OR=0.98, 95% CI=0.53-1.82).

Table 2. Odds ratios with 95% confidence intervals for breast cancer and selective cyclooxygenase-2 (COX-2) inhibitors, and over the counter nonsteroidal anti-inflammatory drugs (OTC NSAIDS)

Compound	Cases	Controls	Multivariate OR[d] (95% CI)
None/Infrequent Use[a]	483	371	1.00
COX-2 Inhibitors[b]	13	61	0.15 (0.08-0.28)
Celecoxib	4	34	0.14 (0.05-0.43)
Rofecoxib	6	26	0.15 (0.06-0.37)
OTC NSAIDs[c]	91	162	0.43 (0.25-0.55)
Aspirin	67	109	0.46 (0.32-0.65)
Ibuprofen/Naproxen	24	53	0.36 (0.21-0.60)
Acetaminophen	24	21	0.98 (0.53-1.82)
Totals	*611*	*615*	

[a] No use of any NSAID or analgesic or infrequent use of no more than one pill per week for less than one year;

[b] COX-2 inhibitors include celecoxib, rofecoxib, valdecoxib, and meloxicam used daily for two years or more.

[c] Over the counter (OTC) NSAIDs/analgesics used at least two times per week for two years or more.

[d] Multivariate odds ratios are adjusted for continuous variables (age and body mass) and categorical variables (parity, menopausal status, family history, smoking, and alcohol intake).

Table 3. Odds ratios for selective COX-2 inhibitors and breast cancer by strata of risk factors or cell membrane receptors

Characteristic	Cases	Controls[a]	Multivariate OR[b] (95% CI)
Menopausal Status			
Premenopausal	251	289	0.12 (0.04-0.45)
Postmenopausal	360	326	0.21 (0.11-0.40)
Family History			
Positive	198	106	0.19 (0.06-0.56)
Negative	413	509	0.14 (0.06-0.30)
Estrogen Receptor			
Positive	226	--	0.24 (0.11-0.51)
Negative	71	--	0.05 (0.01-0.82)
HER-2/*neu*			
Positive	127	--	0.26 (0.06-0.72)
Negative	203	--	0.17 (0.07-0.44)

[a]Odds ratios for cell membrane receptor status (estrogen receptor and HER-2/neu) were calculated using the entire control group of women without breast cancer (n=615).

[b]Multivariate odds ratios are adjusted for continuous variables (age and body mass) and categorical variables (parity, menopausal status, family history, smoking, and alcohol intake).

Table 3 presents risk estimates for COX-2 inhibitors with stratification by menopause, family history, estrogen receptor and HER-2/*neu* status. The observed risk reductions were statistically significant and reasonable consistent across all strata. Cyclooxygenase-2 inhibitors produced significant risk reductions for premenopausal women (OR=0.12), postmenopausal women (OR=0.21), women with a positive family history (OR=0.19), women with a negative family history (OR=0.14), women with estrogen receptor positive tumors (OR=0.24), women with estrogen receptor negative tumors (OR=0.05), women with HER-2/neu positive tumors (OR=0.26), and women with HER-2/neu negative tumors (OR=0.17).

DISCUSSION

The results of this epidemiologic investigation reflect a significant risk reduction in human breast cancer due to intake of selective COX-2 inhibitors. Standard daily dosages of celecoxib (200 mg) or rofecoxib (25 mg) taken for two or more years were associated with an 85% reduction in breast cancer risk. Effects of the selective COX-2 inhibitors were consistent within subgroups of premenopausal and postmenopausal women, and women with and without a family history of breast cancer.

Furthermore, risk reductions were also evident regardless of cell membrane receptors (estrogen receptors and HER-2/neu) measured at the time of diagnosis. Comparator NSAIDs with non-selective COX-2 activity (325 mg aspirin, 200 mg ibuprofen or 250 mg naproxen) also produced significant risk reductions, and it is notable that the effect of ibuprofen, a nonselective NSAID with significant COX-2 activity, was similar to that of selective COX-2 blocking agents. In contrast, acetaminophen did not change the risk of breast cancer.

In general, NSAIDs inhibit cyclooyxgenase which is the key rate-limiting enzyme of prostaglandin biosynthesis [15, 16, 17]. Molecular studies show that the inducible COX-2 gene is over-expressed in human breast cancer and that COX-2 genetic expression in cancer cells is correlated with mutagenesis, mitogenesis, angiogenesis, and deregulation of apoptosis [18, 19, 20]. Over the counter NSAIDs have consistently shown antitumor effects in animal models of carcinogenesis [21], and in recent studies, striking antitumor effects of the specific COX-2 inhibitor, celecoxib, have been observed against breast cancer [22]. In breast cancer cells, COX-2 over-expression is also associated with CYP-19 P-450$_{arom}$ genetic expression and local estrogen biosynthesis [23, 24, 25]. The current study coupled with existing preclinical and molecular evidence suggest that aberrant induction of COX-2 and up-regulation of the prostaglandin cascade play a significant role in mammary carcinogenesis, and that blockade of this process has strong potential for intervention.

Enthusiasm for the use of selective COX-2 blocking agents in the chemoprevention of breast cancer and other malignancies has been tempered by reports of adverse effects on the cardiovascular system leading to the recall of popular anti-arthritic compounds, rofecoxib (Vioxx) and valdecoxib (Bextra). However, such studies involved supra-therapeutic dosages given over long periods of time without consideration of body size or individual differences in metabolism [26].

CONCLUSIONS

We observed a significant reduction in the risk of human breast cancer due to intake of selective COX-2 inhibitors. Chemopreventive effects against breast cancer were associated with recommended daily doses of celecoxib (median dose=200 mg) or rofecoxib (median dose=25 mg) for an average duration of 3.6 years. Notably, selective COX-2 inhibitors (celecoxib and rofecoxib) were only recently approved for use in 1999, and rofecoxib (Vioxx) was withdrawn from the marketplace in 2004. Nevertheless, even in the short window of exposure to these compounds, the selective COX-2 inhibitors produced a significant (85%) reduction in the risk of breast cancer, underscoring their strong potential for breast cancer chemoprevention.

COMPETING INTERESTS

This research was supported in part by a grant from Pfizer, New York, NY, and grant P30 CA16058 from the National Cancer Institute, Bethesda, MD.

AUTHOR'S CONTRIBUTIONS

REH designed and directed the study. JBD coordinated data collection and quality control, and assisted in the interpretation of results. GAA assisted in the analysis and interpretation of results.

ACKNOWLEDGMENTS

The authors thank Elvira M. Garofalo, Program Manager of the James Cancer Mammography Unit, and Julie M. Coursey, Assistant Director of the James Cancer Medical Records Registry, for their assistance in the conduct of this investigation.

REFERENCES

[1]   Couzin J. Withdrawal of Vioxx casts a shadow over COX-2 inhibitors. *Science* 2004, 306, 384-385.
[2]   Couzin J. Clinical Trials: Nail-biting time for trials of drugs. *Science* 2004, 306, 1673-1675.

[3]   Mukherjee D, Nissen SE, Topol EJ. Risk of cardiovascular events associated with selective COX-2 inhibitors. *J. Am. Med. Assoc.* 2001, 286 (8): 954-959.

[4]   Bresalier RS, Sandler RS, Quan H, Bolognese JA, Oxenius B, Horgan K, Lines C, Riddell R, Morton D, Lanas A, Konstam MA, Baron JA. Cardiovascular events associated with rofecoxib in a colorectal adenoma chemoprevention trial. *N. Engl. J. Med. 2005*, 352 (11): 1092-1102.

[5]   Solomon SD, McMurray JJ, Pfeffer MA, Wittes J, Fowler R, Finn P, Anderson WF, Zauber A, Hawk E, Bertagnolli M. Cardiovascular risk associated with celecoxib in a clinical trial for colorectal adenoma prevention. *N. Engl. J. Med.* 2005, 352 (11), 1071-1080.

[6]   White WB, Faich G, Whelton A, Maurath C, Ridge NJ, Verburg KM, Geis GS, Lefkowith JB. Comparison of thromboembolic events in patients treated with celecoxib , a cyclooxygenase-2 specific inhibitor, versus ibuprofen or diclofenac. *Am. J. Cardiol.* 2002, 89 (4): 425-430.

[7]   White WB, Faich G, Borer JS, Makuch RW. Cardiovascular thrombotic events in arthritis trials of the cyclooxygenase-2 inhibitor, celecoxib. *Am. J. Cardiol.* 2003, 92 (4): 411-418.

[8]   Reicin AS, Shapiro D, Sperling RS, Barr E, Yu Q. Comparison of cardiovascular thrombotic events in patients with osteoarthritis treated with rofecoxib versus nonselective nonsteroidal anti-inflammatory drugs (ibuprofen, diclofenac, and nabumetone). *Am. J. Cardiol.* 2002, 89 (2): 204-209.

[9]   Mamdani M, Rochon P, Juurlink DN, Anderson GM, Kopp A, Naglie G, Austin PC, Laupaci A. Effect of selective cyclooxygenase-2 inhibitors and naproxen on short-term risk of acute myocardial infarction in the elderly. *Arch. Intern. Med.* 2003, 163 (4): 481-486.

[10] Shaya FT, Blume SW, Blanchette CM, Weir MR, Mullin CD. Selective cyclooxygenase-2 inhibition and cardiovascular effects: an observational study of a Medicaid population. *Arch. Intern. Med.* 2005, 165 (2): 181-186.

[11] *Cancer Statistics, Incidence and Mortality.* American Cancer Society, 2004.

[12] Harris RE, Beebe-Donk J, Doss H, Burr-Doss D. Aspirin, ibuprofen, and other non-steroidal anti-inflammatory drugs in cancer prevention: a critical review of non-selective COX-2 blockade (Review). *Oncology Reports* 2004, 13: 559-583.

[13] Schlesselman JJ. *Case Control Studies.* Oxford University Press, New York, 1982.

[14] Harrell F. Logistic Regression Procedure. *Statistical Analysis System* (SAS), 2005.

[15] Vane JR. Inhibition of prostaglandin synthesis as a mechanism of action for aspirin-like drugs. *Nature* 1971, 231: 323-235.

[16] Herschman HR. Regulation of prostaglandin synthase-1 and prostaglandin synthase-2. *Cancer and Metas. Rev.* 1994, 13: 241-256.

[17] Hla T and Neilson K. Human cyclooxygenase-2 cDNA. *Proc. Natl. Acad. Sci. USA* 1992, 89: 7384-7388.

[18] 18. Harris RE. Epidemiology of breast cancer and nonsteroidal anti-inflammatory drugs. In: *COX-2 Blockade in Cancer Prevention and Therapy,* Edited by Harris RE. Humana Press, Totowa, NJ, 2002, 57-68.

[19] Parrett ML, Harris RE, Joarder FS, Ross MS, Clausen KP, Robertson FM. Cyclooxygenase-2 gene expression in human breast cancer. *International Journal of Oncology* 1997, 10: 503-507.

[20] 20. Masferrer JL, Leahy KM, Koki AT, Aweifel BS, Settle SL, Woerner BM, Edwards DA, Flickinger AG, Moore RJ, Seibert K. Antiangiogenic and antitumor activities of cyclooxygenase-2 inhibitors. *Cancer Res.* 2000, 60(5): 1306-1311.

[21] Abou-Issa HM, Alshafie GA, Harris RE. Chemoprevention of breast cancer by nonsteroidal anti-inflammatory drugs and selective COX-2 blockade in animals. In: *COX-2 Blockade in Cancer Prevention and Therapy*, Edited by Harris RE. Humana Press, Totowa, NJ, 2002, 85-98.

[22] Harris RE, Alshafie GA, Abou-Issa H, Seibert K. Chemoprevention of breast cancer in rats by Celecoxib, a specific clooygenase-2 (COX-2) inhibitor. *Cancer Res.* 2000, 60: 2101-2103.

[23] Harris RE, Robertson FM, Farrar WB, Brueggemeier RW. Genetic induction and upregulation of cyclooxygenase (COX) and aromatase (CYP-19): an extension of the dietary fat hypothesis of breast cancer. *Medical Hypotheses* 1999, 52 (4): 292-293.

[24] Zhao Y, Agarwal VR, Mendelson CR, Simpson ER. Estrogen biosynthesis proximal to a breast tumor is stimulated by PGE2 via cyclic AMP, leading to activation of promoter II of the CYP19 (aromatase) gene. *Endocrinology* 1996, 137(12): 5739-5742.

[25] Brueggemeier RW, Quinn AL, Parrett ML, Joarder FS, Harris RE, Robertson FM. Correlation of aromatase and cyclooxygenase gene expression in human breast cancer specimens. *Cancer Letters* 1999, 140 (1-2):27-35.

[26] Harris RE. Does the dose make the poison? *Science* 2005 308, 203.

INDEX